Sally Lewis

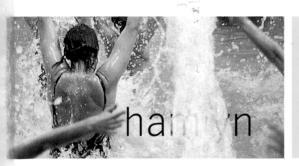

hamlyn

Menopause

Recipes and Advice to Relieve Symptoms

food solutions

Menopause

Recipes and Advice to Relieve Symptoms

food solutions

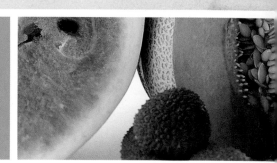

Executive Editor – Jane McIntosh
Senior Editor – Sarah Ford
Editors – Chris McLaughlin and
Lesley Levene
Executive Art Editor – Leigh Jones
Book Design – Birgit Eggers
Picture Research – Zoe Holterman
Production – Lucy Woodhead

Copyright © Octopus Publishing
Group Ltd 2001
ISBN 0 600 60298 2

First published
in Great Britain in 2001
by Hamlyn, an imprint of
Octopus Publishing Group Ltd,
2–4 Heron Quays, London E14 4JP

A CIP catalogue record for this book is
available from the British Library

Printed and bound in China
10 9 8 7 6 5 4 3 2 1

Distributed in the United States
by Sterling Publishing Co., Inc.
387 Park Avenue South, New York, NY10016–8810

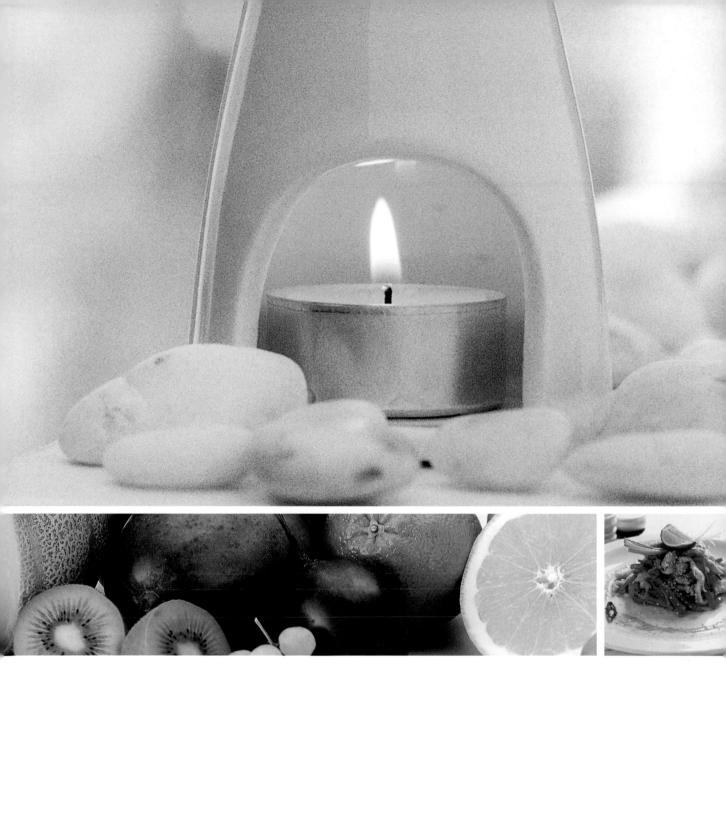

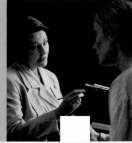
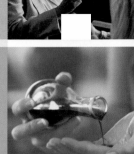
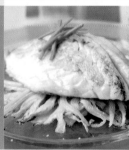
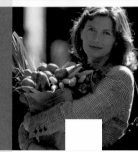
contents

menopause

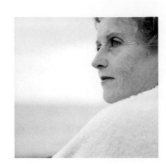

LEFT: In many parts of the world post-menopausal women are revered for their wisdom and experience. This attitude is gradually returning to Western societies.

Virtually all women regard the menopause as a time of significant change – physically, psychologically and emotionally – and many dread its onset. Although a woman's body does undergo important changes during and following her menopause, this does not have to be a negative experience. Many women find fresh sources of enjoyment and satisfaction in this new phase of life and are able to manage menopausal symptoms with varying combinations of conventional and complementary treatment and changes to their lifestyle and diet.

In Western societies, which put a high value on youth, the menopause is associated with the ageing process and so all too often is seen as the beginning of an inevitable decline. At one time it was a subject shrouded in secrecy and hedged around with taboos, and even now many people wrongly believe that once a woman's menopause is over, she inevitably becomes wrinkled, dried up and bent. However, in parts of the world where older people are respected and even revered, a post-menopausal woman may be treated quite differently and regarded as a fount of wisdom and useful experience.

Both medical scientists and, equally important, women themselves are now discovering more about the changes that take place around the time of the menopause and how best to handle them. Virtually every week, if not every day, an item appears somewhere in the media about new findings, treatments, diet or other self-help approaches that minimize the ill-effects of the hormonal changes that underlie the menopause. Although they are not the result of any illness, many of the common symptoms associated with the menopause are easier to deal with and alleviate when you understand what is causing them and what you yourself can do about them. The more women understand the changes that are taking place in their bodies, and the possible consequences, the easier it is to approach them in a positive and constructive way.

Recognizing and taking steps to alleviate physical symptoms are, however, not always sufficient by themselves. For many women, such physical problems are less significant than the sense that the menopause signals the end of their femininity, their sexual appeal and interest, and

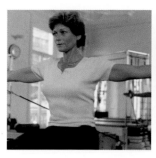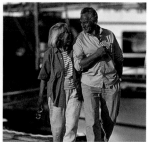

LEFT: **Maintaining good health and a positive attitude are the main ingredients to leading a fulfilling life throughout and after the menopause.**

that henceforth they will become increasingly 'invisible' to the rest of the world. It can seem as if loss of fertility means that you are no longer a real woman and the best years of your life are over. There is no reason to accept any of these outdated attitudes, and the more positive you are able to be about what you want to do with the rest of your life the better. It is important to realize that your body does not age more rapidly after the menopause and that you can do a great deal to maintain your health and fitness for many years to come. The menopause does not signal the end of your sex life either: many women find that not having to worry about contraception liberates their libido and their enjoyment of sex actually increases. If you see the menopause as the beginning of a new phase in your life rather than as an end, you will improve your enjoyment of the years that follow as much as the ones that went before.

The way the menopause affects you and how you deal with it will be unique to you. Some women have few symptoms or only very minor ones; others may need conventional and/or complementary treatment to alleviate troublesome symptoms. The various forms of complementary therapy not only help with these, but also improve your state of mind, easing tension and lifting your mood. Changes to your lifestyle can enhance your health and sense of well-being whether or not you have any symptoms, especially if you make sure you are following the right kind of diet. There is evidence that certain foods improve hormonal balance, as well as contributing to the efficient functioning of your immune system and keeping bodily functions in good working order.

The important thing to bear in mind is that you are in control: you can choose what steps to take and decide which is the right road for you. This book aims to help you make these choices by providing information about all the options available. Whatever you do, you will benefit from thinking about your diet and making adjustments to ensure that you are getting all the nutrients you need. Once you have decided what changes to make, you will find plenty of inspiration in the recipes in this book. Take your pick from the delicious dishes on offer, confident that the meals you make will not only enhance your health but taste wonderful too!

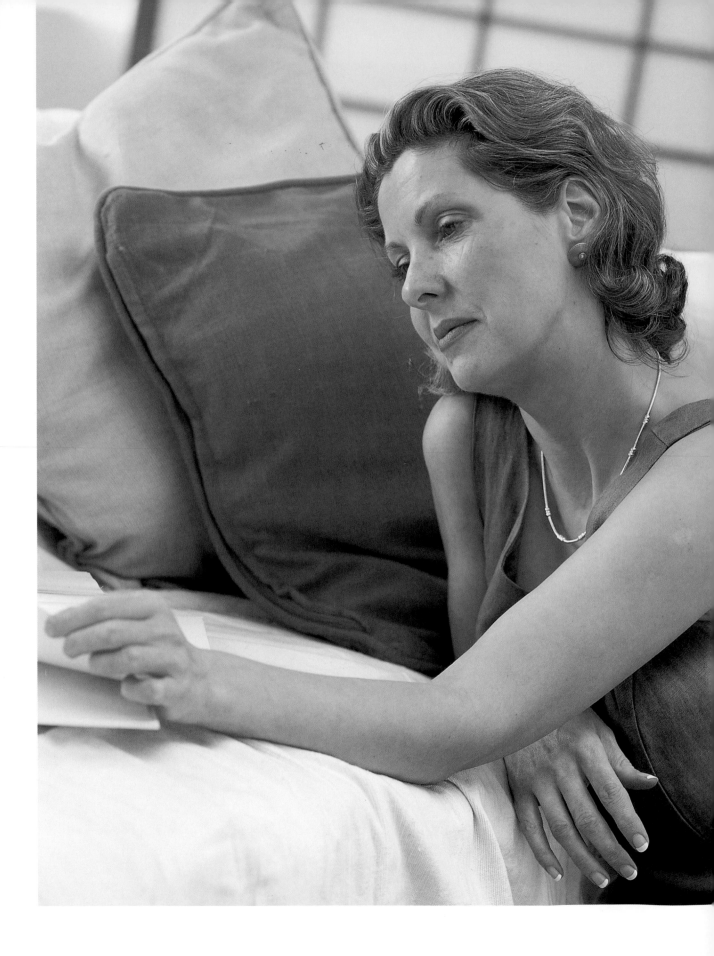

Before considering the enormous **range of symptoms, both physical and psychological**, which can be associated with the menopause, it is important to stress that there may be many other factors which could affect a woman's health and mental well-being at this period of her life. Friends and family – and even some doctors – may be inclined to ascribe any complaints to the menopause, whether or not they are truly related. The other important point to bear in mind is that the list of symptoms that follows includes everything which might conceivably be related to the hormonal changes surrounding the menopause, even though in reality no one will experience all of them and some women will have very few if any, or only very minor ones.

This chapter describes the range of physical, emotional and psychological symptoms that menopausal women may experience in different degrees and **explains what causes them**.

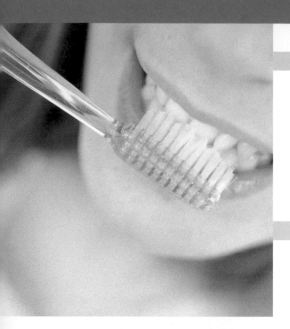

ABOVE: Hormone changes can, in extreme cases, result in gum and teeth infections, so dental hygiene is important.

collagen and elastin

These are proteins which make up the connective tissue throughout the body, providing strength and elasticity in joints, muscles and skin, and the tough fibres which hold organs and joints in place. However, the cells that generate these proteins are sensitive to oestrogen and become less active and effective as the level drops. The resultant effects on collagen and elastin fibres can have repercussions throughout the body.

JOINT PAINS

Muscles and joints may become stiff and painful as hormonal changes cause them to lose some of their strength and elasticity. As well as the lower back, the wrists, knees and ankles tend to be the main problem areas as far as pain is concerned. Again, there may be other reasons for such symptoms and you should talk to your doctor if you experience pain that is more than trivial or short-term.

SKIN

Like other tissues elsewhere in the body, the skin will react to the decline in oestrogen. It becomes thinner, less taut and elastic, and wrinkles start to look more noticeable. Usually it becomes drier, blood vessels beneath its surface are more obvious and visible, and bruising occurs more easily. Some women develop patches of brown pigmentation or find their skin is increasingly itchy. In some cases, this may be a sign of a condition known as formication, so called because it feels like ants (*formicae* in Latin) crawling over the skin. Its exact cause is not known, but it usually disappears without treatment eventually.

NAILS

Finger- and toenails become brittle and split or break easily; some women develop noticeable white spots on their nails.

HAIR

The decline in oestrogen slows down the growth rate of hair, which will tend to become thinner, drier and more fragile. Most women notice that their hair gradually loses its former shine and bounce and some develop dandruff for the first time.

MOUTH AND GUMS

Some people are bothered by cracking skin at the corners of the mouth and by frequent mouth ulcers that heal very slowly. The mouth sometimes feels uncomfortably dry and the gums get soft and puffy. If the gums start to bleed, infection can become a real problem for both gums and, eventually, teeth. Also, as the gums start to shrink, tooth roots may become exposed, hence the expression 'long in the tooth' to describe an older person.

MASCULINIZATION

As oestrogen declines, the effects of androgens become more pronounced. All women produce these male hormones as well as the female ones, but androgen production continues even once the ovaries have stopped secreting oestrogen. Relatively high levels of male hormones encourage the growth of hair on the face and sometimes elsewhere on the upper body and can also result in the voice getting deeper.

WEIGHT GAIN

Almost all women gain weight after the menopause and find that their shape alters as the fat settles in different places. These are natural consequences of lower oestrogen levels and a tendency for the metabolism – the rate at which the body consumes 'fuel' – to slow as you get older. However, there is something to be said in favour of a little extra weight: although your ovaries stop secreting oestrogen the fat cells continue to do so, so carrying a little extra fat – say 4.5kg (10lb) – will increase your oestrogen level and help to counter the effects of its decline.

PROLAPSE

In some women, the weakening of the fibres in the soft tissue holding various internal organs (such as the uterus, bladder, urethra and rectum) in place may cause them to drop. Such problems usually affect women whose internal supports have been weakened as a result of giving birth.

BELOW: Osteoporosis is a weakening of the bones due to a decline in hormone levels in older women.

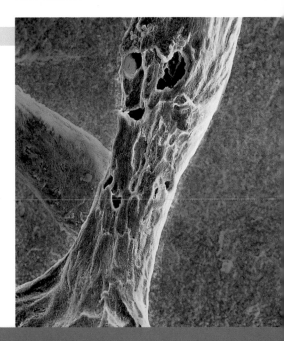

OSTEOPOROSIS

This is a serious condition that affects mainly post-menopausal women and means that bones break easily after minor falls or stresses; it can also result in the upper spine becoming deformed into a 'dowager's hump'. In healthy people, bone is lost and replaced on a regular basis, the whole process under the control of hormones, including oestrogen. As hormone levels decline, bone is not replaced as quickly and the result is a weakening of the bones. Spaces develop within the bones, giving them a sponge-like appearance and making them brittle. Most at risk are small, slim women whose bone mass is lower than average, poorly nourished women, heavy smokers, women with medical conditions such as rheumatoid arthritis, amenorrhoea (absence of periods) or an over-active thyroid, and those on medical treatments such as steroid drugs. In addition, women who have never taken much exercise of the weight-bearing kind and those whose diet

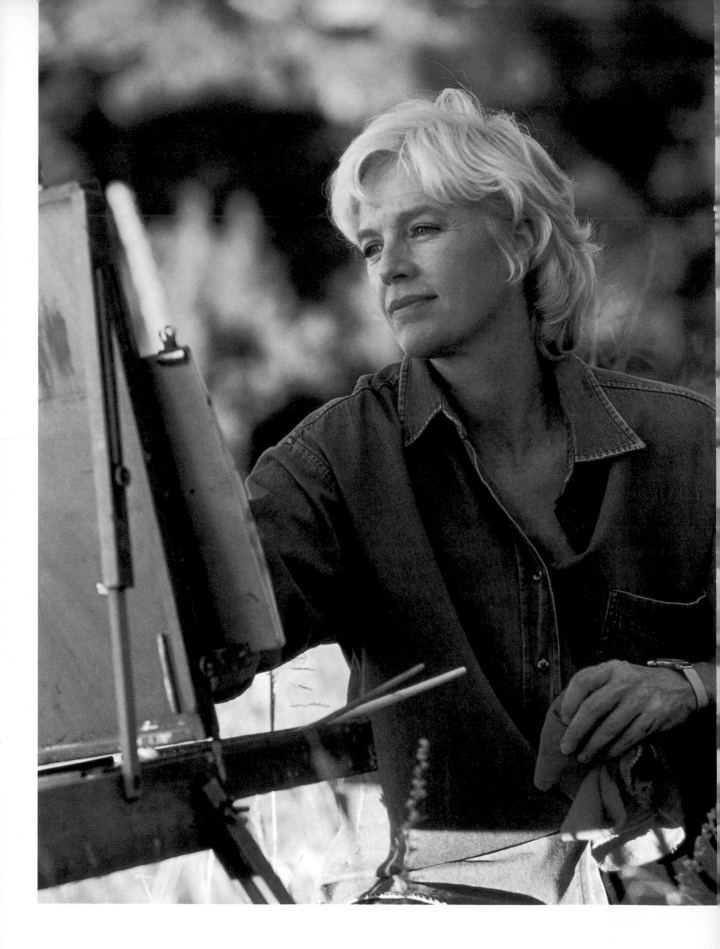

For many women, the prospect of the oncoming menopause is daunting, if not depressing. Fear of the impending **physical and emotional changes** and not knowing what to expect are often exacerbated by gloomy or alarming stories in the media. Yet there may be no need to anticipate the menopause with trepidation. Change is part of life and something everyone has to face at certain points, whether it is through choice or circumstance or a combination of both.

The menopause can, if you let it, be turned into an **opportunity for reflection and awareness**. You will benefit from finding time to look back on what you have achieved so far and to think about what you want in the future and how you plan to make the most of life from now on. **By focusing on yourself and your future**, you make it possible to take responsibility for what happens in your life, to be open to new and enjoyable experiences.

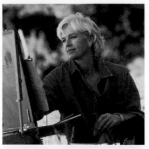

helping yourself

a positive approach

Many women today will live a third of their total life-span after the menopause – an experience that was comparatively rare in earlier generations. We all know that our bodies change as we get older, but for most women the menopause begins around the same time that they start to notice visible signs of ageing. Yet this does not automatically imply that you will be in need of medical attention. Many women go through the menopause with few or no serious symptoms or problems, although some of course may have more than their fair share of troubles. No one can predict exactly what will happen, but your approach to this new stage of your life will have an important influence on how you deal with the changes that are taking place in your body. A positive outlook, an ability to adapt and making time to take a fresh look at your lifestyle will all help you to cope. Some changes are likely to be beyond your control, such as children leaving home or changes in your role at work or your responsibilities towards ageing parents, and you may well wonder what you should do for the best. Taking steps to make sure you remain as healthy as possible and looking after your own emotional and psychological wellbeing will improve your chances of handling whatever should come along in this next phase of your life.

a good social life

If family life with your partner and children has been the mainstay of your life up to now, you can easily feel isolated and bereft when the time comes for your offspring to move away. Some women feel a sense of loss when the cessation of their periods means they have to accept that children are no longer even a theoretical possibility; others are simply thankful that contraception is no longer important. Natural concerns about ageing and the increased risk of health problems such as osteoporosis and heart disease can, to a considerable extent, be alleviated by following the advice in this book. Depression can sometimes accompany the menopause, but, as well as seeking any treatment that is necessary, making sure you have a good social network can do much to keep it at bay.

It is important to have friends with whom you can share the bad times as well as the good. Having friends who encourage you to join in social activities can help you to feel positive about yourself and keep up vital links with the outside world. Those women who do experience troublesome menopausal symptoms often find them more manageable if they can share their experiences with others who are going or have gone through something similar.

Many women find that changing home circumstances mean they now have more time and energy to take up new activities and join groups where they make new friends. Plenty of organizations now target those aged over 50, but even if you are not sure whether these are for you, the option is always there and may be worth exploring. Try not to rule out any possibilities, especially if you have previously been very much involved in family life and have had little incentive or opportunity to develop separate personal friendships and activities up until now. This can be a good time to follow up an interest you have always had but for which you have never previously had time or energy to spare. Many women find that they enter a new, creative phase of life after the menopause and develop hitherto unexplored talents in spheres such as writing, painting, the decorative arts or dance, for example.

The opportunity to put yourself and your personal needs first can be a new and very rewarding experience. Wherever you happen to live, you will surely find many activities on offer, some of which will be right for you. There are classes in just about everything you can think of, as well as books, cassettes and videos that can introduce you to a whole range of intriguing possibilities. In the following pages, you will find some suggestions which can serve as a starting point while you consider all the possible options. In particular, you might think of exploring some of the different relaxation techniques and yoga, which have much to offer in terms of improved mental and physical well-being and easing minor menopausal symptoms.

relaxation

Many women who practise relaxation sessions on a daily basis have found that these help to ease hot flushes. With some claiming a reduction in symptoms of up to half, it really is worth finding the time to try the techniques for yourself. Contrary to a commonly held belief, there is much more to relaxation than simply sitting in a comfortable chair with a magazine or watching TV. The techniques have to be learned and practised, and although some master them relatively easily, others find it takes time to learn how to do so. Fortunately, there is a lot of help available: you can buy cassette and video tapes if you prefer to learn at home or you can join a class, where you will also have the opportunity to meet new people and an incentive to attend on a regular basis.

One of the most important benefits of learning how to relax properly is that you can use the techniques to counter the ill-effects of stress. Despite its bad reputation, stress does have some positive aspects, as it helps to galvanize us into taking necessary action when required, but too much or constant stress can deplete the body's resources and have a detrimental effect on health. When you are feeling completely stressed out and about to explode, trying to make yourself relax can be a real challenge. However, once you have mastered the techniques you will be

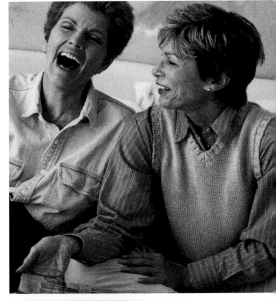

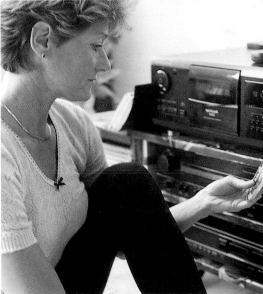

TOP: Keeping up with old friends or making new ones is vital for a healthy outlook.

ABOVE: Relaxation techniques can reduce hot flushes – join a relaxation class or use videos, cassettes and CDs at home.

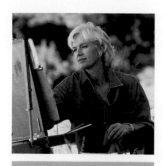

aware of when you are experiencing stress and so be better able to deal with it before it gets out of hand. Developing an awareness of your body and the signals it sends out makes stressful situations much easier to deal with. Relaxation techniques have the effect of slowing a rapid heartbeat, regulating breathing and controlling the metabolic rate. They also reduce your adrenaline levels, which rise when you are under stress, allow the immune system to function more effectively and can ease related symptoms such as headaches and migraines.

simple relaxation

There are many different techniques but one simple tried and tested method is consciously to tense and relax every muscle in the body in turn.

Choose a quiet room where you will not be disturbed; if necessary take the phone off the hook and disconnect the door bell.

1	Lie or sit comfortably, close your eyes and become aware of your body. Try not to think about any worries or tasks that need doing and concentrate your attention on your body and, in particular, on any areas of physical tension.
2	Breathe in deeply and slowly through your nose, then exhale slowly through your mouth.
3	Allow your tongue to come away from the roof of your mouth and relax the lips and surrounding muscles as you continue to breathe in and out.
4	Focus on your feet, tightening your toes as you inhale, then hold for a count of five. Exhale through your mouth, releasing your toes.
5	Now work up through your body, tightening each set of muscles in turn, starting with your calves, then releasing them after a count of five.
6	Continue to tense and release each major set of muscles until you have worked on those in your neck and face.
7	Now continue to breathe deeply and slowly for a few minutes before opening your eyes and stretching your whole body. You should feel relaxed and refreshed.

VISUALIZATION

An alternative name for this technique is 'creative imagery', because it involves summoning up mental images that encourage a sense of relaxation and tranquillity. Positive visualization can be associated with achieving a specific goal – which is why competitive athletes often use it as part of their mental preparation and motivational training. Even if you have no interest in scoring goals or breaking sprint records, you can use the same method to help you overcome particular worries and fears. Before you begin, select an image that is associated in your mind with calm and relaxation such as a beautiful sunset or a peaceful beach or country scene.

simple visualization

Choose a quiet, comfortable location where you will not be disturbed and find a comfortable place to sit or lie down.

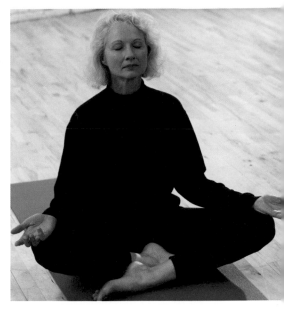

ABOVE: Meditation, if performed every day, can help to lower stress-related symptoms including high blood pressure, headaches and migraines.

Close your eyes and breathe slowly and deeply in through your nose and out through your mouth.	1
Try to create an image of your chosen scene in your mind and hold it there.	2
Use your other senses to fill in the picture: smell the flowers in the garden, for example, or listen to the sound of the waves on the shore.	3
Keep your breathing regular and relaxed and keep pushing aside any intrusive thoughts, concentrating on the mental image.	4
Stay in this place as long as you like, then gently bring yourself back to the present. Imagine yourself leaving the scene slowly and coming back to reality, then open your eyes, giving yourself time to readjust.	5

MEDITATION

This is similar to relaxation and is another way of freeing your mind from distressing or worrying thoughts. The main difference is that it uses a sound or short phrase as a mental focus point to clear away intrusive thoughts. With practice, mediation can achieve a very deep level of relaxation. There is some evidence that daily meditation can help to lower raised blood pressure and ease headaches, migraine symptoms and other stress-related problems. There are many different approaches to meditation and the technique is best learned from a teacher or by following the instructions on a cassette, but you can try at home by selecting your word

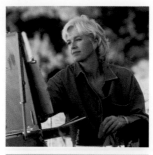

helping yourself

or phrase, then focusing on it in the same way as in the visualization technique explained on page 27. Instead of conjuring the image, you simply repeat the words (or mantra) whenever unwanted thoughts intrude.

YOGA

You don't have to be a contortionist or even particularly supple to learn simple yoga, and everyone can benefit from practising this ancient Eastern art. If at all possible, you should learn from a qualified teacher, as it is difficult to know whether you are doing the movements correctly on your own. However, it is easy to find beginners' classes almost everywhere and experienced teachers encourage everyone to work at their own pace and level without any element of competition. Yoga offers both physical and mental benefits: it stretches the body and clears the mind, promoting a sense of calm and peace. As you become more proficient, you will find that your body becomes stronger and more flexible and you cope more easily with mental stress and upset. Advanced yoga involves a profound mental discipline, but most beginners' classes in the West concentrate on Hatha yoga, which involves practising breathing (*pranayama*), poses (*asanas*) and meditation (*dhyana*). The breathing exercises are important because they improve physical energy and vitality as well as toning the circulation and strengthening the lungs. Yoga is beneficial for women of menopausal age because you work at your own pace, progressing to the more difficult moves without placing undue stress on your body. It can help to ease symptoms such as headaches, hot flushes, depression and anxiety and improves overall muscular tone and flexibility.

THE ALEXANDER TECHNIQUE

This is a way of re-educating the body out of bad habits of movement and posture that have been acquired over the years. Originally developed by Frederick Alexander, it involves using a combination of gentle instruction and guided movement which is designed to help you to rediscover your natural physical poise, grace and freedom of movement and so eliminate postural strains and symptoms such as pain and tension arising from them. It is possible to learn the basics from a book or a video, but it is far better to attend classes with a teacher who can tailor the techniques to your personal needs and ensure that you are moving correctly.

exercise

The very word is enough to elicit a groan from people who have done virtually no exercise for years and find even thinking about the prospect daunting if not exhausting. Yet the benefits are very real and can hardly

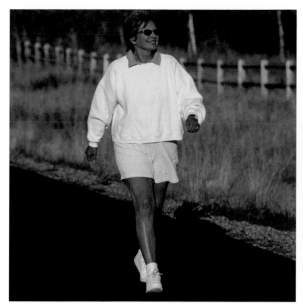

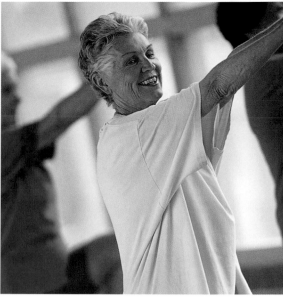

be over-stressed. This is particularly true for women around the time of the menopause, because taking the right kind of exercise not only boosts general health but is also very effective in controlling weight gain, lifting depression, relieving anxiety, alleviating insomnia and improving self-esteem.

Weight-bearing exercise is especially important in this phase of your life, because it helps to strengthen bones and stave off osteoporosis (see page 19). Walking, jogging, racket sports, dancing, aerobics, skating and skipping all qualify as weight-bearing and it is literally never too late to begin and gain the benefits. As well as increasing your energy and vitality, exercise is great for lifting your mood and keeping depression at bay. In purely physical terms, regular exercise that works up a light sweat and leaves you breathing a little faster than usual will tone up your whole cardiovascular system, leaving you less vulnerable to diseases that affect your heart, blood vessels and lungs, as well as firming your muscles and other soft tissue.

When you have been exercising on a regular basis for just a few weeks, you will notice that you are able to cope better with stress, and your improved fitness and sense of wellbeing will give you an enormous lift. Some of the psychological benefits of regular exercise are thought to be due to the fact that it stimulates the production of brain chemicals called endorphins, sometimes known as 'feel-good chemicals'. These create a feeling of calm and alertness and are very effective at countering any tendency to low moods.

Other hormones stimulated by exercise can actually have the effect of making you feel less hungry than you might expect afterwards, and many people say they feel less tempted by 'unhealthy' foods like sweet and fatty fare. In fact, the best fuel for exercise is complex carbohydrates such as pasta, which release a steady supply of energy in the form of

ABOVE LEFT: Even a brisk walk every day that leaves you a little breathless will work wonders with your physical and mental wellbeing.

ABOVE RIGHT: Aerobics classes, like any other form of weight-bearing exercise, will strengthen bones and protect you against osteoporosis – and they can be great fun.

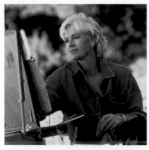

helping yourself

blood glucose. They are also the best way to top up your energy levels afterwards. Make sure to replace lost fluids by drinking plenty of water both during and after strenuous exercise.

The trouble with exercise is that you can't store it up – you have to keep on doing it or the benefits will be lost before very long. However, the good news is that once you have felt and seen those benefits for yourself, you won't want to stop, even if you have been a couch potato all your life up until now.

BONE HEALTH

The main reason why weight-bearing exercise is so vital is, as we have seen, the role it plays in improving bone density and so lessening the risk of osteoporosis developing following the menopause. In fact, the earlier in life you begin taking this type of exercise, the greater the beneficial effects, as it will boost the peak bone density, which is usually reached around the age of 35. Earlier generations of women rarely needed to make any deliberate effort to exercise because physical activity was a normal part of their lives: they walked, sometimes long distances, to school, work and the shops, often carrying heavy bags, and probably did hard physical labour in the kitchen and garden as well. Today, when most people normally travel by car or public transport rather than walking and have access to all kinds of labour-saving devices at home, we have to make a special effort to build exercise into our lives unless we are naturally sporty types.

By placing physical stress on our bodies through exercise, we not only encourage the process of building bone but also increase the amount of 'pull' exerted on bones by the muscles attached to them, so further encouraging bone health by making bone-building cells more active. The loss of oestrogen following the menopause accelerates natural bone loss, which begins slowly in the late thirties, so that by the time women reach their mid-sixties, many of them are increasingly vulnerable to fractures because their bones have lost so much of their former strength.

Before we consider specific types of exercise, it is worth bearing in mind that even small increases in physical activity can help: walking rather than driving to the shops or to work, using stairs rather than lifts or escalators, or just giving the dog a slightly longer walk each day. If you have never gone in for exercise, you might start by taking a short but brisk daily walk, increasing your speed and distance as your fitness improves. You should also check with your doctor before you take up exercise in earnest to see whether there is any activity you should avoid because of existing health problems, or indeed any type which would be particularly beneficial.

Although you need to think about taking exercise for health reasons, you are unlikely to stick with it for long unless you choose an activity you

BELOW: During and after exercise, be sure to drink plenty of water to replace lost fluids.

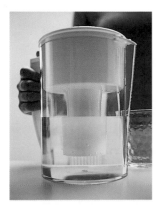

the aims of exercise

Basically, you need to consider three aspects of fitness: increasing strength, stamina and flexibility.

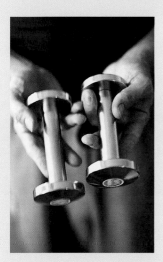

ABOVE: Small weights can help to build upper body strength, improving posture and making daily tasks easier.

→ **strength** – this does not mean developing muscles like Miss Universe; in fact, to do so is not easy and requires a specific training programme. Becoming strong is something entirely different and, in the majority of cases, means paying particular attention to your upper body. Building up strength in this area will not only improve your posture but make many everyday tasks much easier – for example, lifting and carrying heavy items, gardening and decorating will all feel much less of an effort.

→ **stamina** – this term actually refers to the amount of oxygen supplied to your muscles by the action of your heart and lungs. When you are unfit, you will find yourself breathless and tired after a short burst of effort such as running for a bus or swimming one length of a pool. You will take a while to recover afterwards and you may just assume this is inevitable as you get older, but that is not the case. You can improve your stamina at any age by taking the kind of exercise that develops the heart and lungs. This means aerobic work: in other words, activity that involves increased uptake of oxygen, such as running, jogging or dancing. Once you have begun exercising, your stamina will increase relatively quickly. Even people who have had a heart attack can recover sufficiently to run a marathon, although, of course, this isn't a suitable or even desirable goal for most people. Walking and jogging cost nothing and can be done in the open air in the right climate, but wherever you are there are likely to be exercise classes of various types or a gym within easy reach and many organize special classes for the over-fifties if that appeals.

→ **flexibility** – this does not mean the ability to do the splits or move like a ballet dancer. Rather it is about keeping the joints mobile and moving freely, and countering any tendency to stiffness that comes with increasing years. Exercise keeps the muscles around joints strong and flexible and also reduces vulnerability to injury when you happen to move suddenly or awkwardly. Anyone can do daily stretching exercises at home or, if you prefer to join a class, consider taking up yoga, tai chi, chi kung or pilates, which are gentle but very effective.

enjoy. If cost is a factor in your decision, think about something that involves relatively little expense, such as walking or jogging, although you will need to invest in the right footwear. You do not need expensive, high-fashion trainers but you do need shoes designed to protect your feet and knees by cushioning the impact with the ground; your nearest sports equipment shops should be able to advise you if necessary. Some people find that paying out for membership of a gym or sports centre gives them the incentive they need to go regularly, and although the initial outlay can be quite high, the cost per visit often works out to be quite reasonable if you use the facilities several times a week. Whatever you choose, aim to build up to five sessions per week of around 30 minutes each; you can do the same thing every time or opt for a mix of different activities to gain maximum benefits.

take your pick

The best exercise is something you enjoy and so will continue to do on a regular basis. Try to include some of the following weight-bearing types, but the most important thing is to make a start.

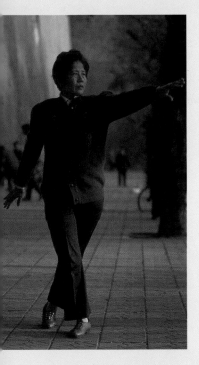

ABOVE: Tai chi requires coordination, concentration and flexibility.

→ **walking** – much under-estimated as a form of exercise, it is easy and free. All you have to do is rouse yourself to go out and walk briskly for at least 30 minutes. Aim to go fast enough to be slightly out of breath but still able to hold a conversation; any slower and you will not be making any beneficial impact on your heart and lungs.

→ **jogging** – start slowly if you have never done it before and do a few minutes' stretching prior to setting off (and again afterwards) to prevent the build-up of lactic acid, which will otherwise leave you with sore muscles. You could begin by alternating walking with jogging until you get a bit fitter. It will alleviate the boredom and encourage you to continue if you can persuade someone else to join you.

→ **rebounder** – most sports shops stock these mini-trampolines, which are especially useful if the weather discourages outdoor exercise. Bouncing works your heart and lungs without causing any stress on joints in the lower limbs.

→ **aerobics** – you should have no trouble finding a local class, but make sure that the teacher is qualified and avoid anyone who adopts a 'no gain without pain' approach. If you're unfit, go for low-impact aerobics, which is less physically demanding than the high-impact kind. Alternatively, you can choose one of the many aerobics videos to follow at home.

→ **tai chi** – this stylized system of movements, which originated in China, requires concentration and controlled breathing. The movements are slow and subtle and are designed to coordinate body, mind and spirit, so they can be good for reducing stress and encouraging relaxation.

→ **yoga** – this is very useful for improving overall strength and flexibility through postures and stretching, and most classes involve elements of relaxation and controlled breathing. Good for newcomers to exercise, although advanced yoga is physically demanding.

→ **pilates** – a system of coordinated exercise and breathing that is especially good for toning muscles and improving posture while encouraging mental and spiritual calm and harmony.

a healthy sex life

There are many reasons why your sex life may go off the boil around the time of the menopause but it is certainly not inevitable. Plenty of couples continue to have a good physical relationship into their seventies and beyond, so you should not assume that if yours is disappointing there is nothing to be done. The decline may relate to a loss of libido, physical pain or discomfort, problems within your relationship, a loss of confidence in your own sexual attractiveness or even simple boredom – alone or in combination.

Loss of libido can be a consequence of declining oestrogen or sometimes because sexual intercourse is uncomfortable or painful because of vaginal dryness and lack of lubrication. HRT will help with both, and a lubricating jelly will help with dryness. Exercise that tones up the circulation will increase the blood supply to the genital area and you should also make sure your diet includes an adequate supply of vitamins and minerals to keep the tissues healthy and maintain your energy levels. Pelvic floor exercises (see below) will help tighten the vagina if practised frequently and regularly.

If you are concerned about the changes affecting you both mentally and physically around the time of your menopause, try to be as open as you can with your partner about what is happening and how you feel. Changing when and where you make love may revive your interest if sex has become too much of a routine. There is no reason why you should have sex only at night in the bedroom, even if that is what you have always done previously. When intercourse does not appeal, see whether your partner would be willing to try a massage session using aromatherapy oils; this can be very relaxing and a nice way of showing your love even when you don't feel like sex. If both of you like the idea of something a little different, consider creating a special atmosphere with candles, soft music, champagne in bed or even something more outrageous... Remember, you don't have to be serious and if things don't quite work at least you can laugh together.

Sex is good for you. It is relaxing, it releases hormones that lift your mood and it helps sustain a feeling of closeness with your partner. While HRT is often effective at treating problems such as loss of libido, taking it can sometimes create the impression that the menopause is an illness and thus undermine a woman's confidence in her sexuality. In fact, many women find that their interest in sex increases after the menopause: they no longer worry about contraception or being interrupted by the children and have more time and energy. Although oestrogen levels decline, the relative increase in levels of the male hormone testosterone can result in an increased sex drive. Of course, a man may also have difficulties with sex for either physical or psychological reasons. Being open with one another is a good first step, and if necessary, a woman may need to encourage her partner to consult his doctor about a problem such as erectile dysfunction, as this can often be treated effectively.

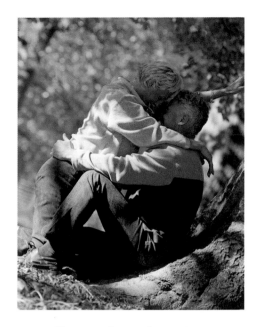

ABOVE: Many couples continue to have a good physical relationship in later life. Maintaining intimacy is a good way to show love for your partner.

simple pelvic exercises

→ Each time you go to the loo, try stopping the urine flow midstream; the muscles you use to do this are your pelvic floor muscles.

→ When you have stopped the flow, hold this position for a count of three before releasing the flow.

→ Once you can do this, practise drawing up these muscles at other times, hold for a count of five, then release slowly.

→ Do this exercise whenever you think of it, but no fewer than ten times every day.

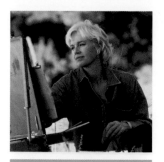

helping yourself

caring for your body

All women should develop breast awareness and become familiar with the way their breasts look and feel. This makes it more likely that you will notice any changes and get them professionally checked early on. Most women have strong feelings about their breasts – whether they love or hate them – and these feelings are usually an important element in the way they see themselves and their self-esteem. Few women have breasts that are exactly the same size and shape as one another, and many feel that their breasts are too large or too small. Apart from surgery, however, there is little that can be done to change this. Breasts have no muscle, but the pectoral muscles underneath can be strengthened and developed by exercise so as to provide better support. Breasts are supplied by blood from the major arteries that also supply the chest wall; they are drained through a network of veins.

During the menopause breasts can shrink or become slack as the oestrogen that stimulates the tissues declines and the breast tissue becomes less dense. Some women, on the other hand, find their breasts get bigger as the number of fat cells increases in response to hormonal changes.

It is advisable to examine your breasts monthly, preferably during the week after your period has ended if you are still menstruating. Lumps and bumps are quite common in the week before menstruation, although they tend to disappear after the menopause as oestrogen is no longer stimulating the milk ducts in preparation for pregnancy and birth.

breast awareness

1	Stand facing the mirror, arms by your side, undressed to the waist. Look at your breasts and note any visible change. If you are looking at them for the first time, just take note of the way they look so you can compare it to next time.
2	Raise both arms behind your head, look at your breasts, then do the same thing again turning first to one side and then to the other.
3	Turn to face the mirror, place both hands on your hips and push hard. This should tighten your chest muscles. Note the shape of each breast from every angle.
4	With a soapy hand, in the bath or shower, pass the flat of your fingers all over each breast without squeezing or prodding, using the right hand for the left breast and vice versa. Remember to include the 'tail' of each breast that runs into the armpit and the area below the collarbone. Look for any lumpiness; any dent or dimple in the skin when you lift the arm; any change in skin colour or texture; an inverted nipple; or any discharge or bleeding. Look for any other changes; be aware of what is normal for you.

Skin gradually loses elasticity around the menopause and over subsequent years due to declining oestrogen levels, and this is often most obvious on the face. You develop wrinkles and your skin is likely to become much drier. Using moisturizer every day will help but it cannot prevent the underlying changes. The skin also loses its tone because the supporting tissues weaken once your oestrogen levels drop (see Collagen and elastin, page 18). You may also notice small 'liver spots' or moles appearing.

HRT prevents these changes and many women see an improvement in their skin after taking it for a relatively short time. You can slow the progress of this deterioration somewhat by good skin care – especially thorough cleansing, frequent moisturizing, drinking plenty of water and protecting your skin from damaging ultraviolet sunlight. Cover up as much as possible and always use sun-protection preparations, even on cloudy days. Beauty treatments such as facials, massage, face masks, electro-desiccation and chemical skin-peeling can improve the appearance of the skin, although they will not affect the underlying processes responsible for causing the changes. Smoking makes wrinkles worse and alcohol can cause broken blood vessels on the face; on the other hand, a healthy diet rich in vitamins and minerals will help nourish the skin.

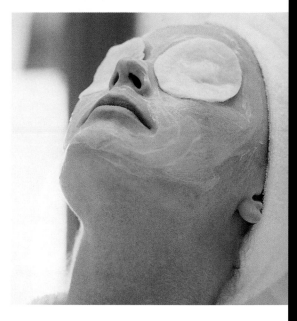

ABOVE: Taking good care of your skin with regular beauty treatments will greatly repay the effort spent.

simple facial exercises

Spend a minute on each exercise, practising in front of a mirror to begin with.

→ **Eyes** – to tone the surrounding muscles and lessen the appearance of crow's feet:
- Stare hard but with your eyes closed; you will feel tension in the surrounding area.
- Keeping your eyes shut, tighten them, screwing up and 'looking' inward with your eyes crossed. Hold for a few seconds.
- Open your eyes as wide as you can and stare at a fixed point.
- Blink rapidly ten to fifteen times, then close your eyes until you feel that the pupils have returned to normal.

→ **Laughter lines** – to ease lines running from the outer edge of the nostrils to the corners of the mouth:
- Raise the corners of your mouth and upper lip, stretching the top lip up and over the teeth while opening your mouth about 2cm. Keep your mouth and neck muscles relaxed, but feel the tension in your cheek pads.
- Suck the air into one cheek, then move it to the opposite one. Suck the air into both cheeks and the area above your top lip. 'Chew' the air. Repeat five to ten times.
- Pursing the lips gently, open them about 1cm, as if blowing bubbles, and exhale gently.

→ **Frown lines** – to tone the muscles that create the vertical lines between your eyebrows:
- Frown hard, then relax the muscles.
- Put your three middle fingers from each hand on the outer edge of each eyebrow and frown. Feel the pull on your fingers.
- Close your eyes and relax the muscles by vibrating your fingertips lightly over your forehead.

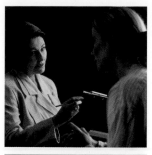

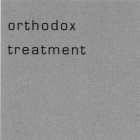

orthodox
treatment

hormone replacement therapy

There are so many myths and half-truths relating to HRT, it is important to understand what it can and cannot do. It certainly cannot reverse or halt the ageing process or make a woman look years younger than her real age. However, if it eliminates problems such as hot flushes and broken nights, it can restore a woman's natural energy and vitality so that she feels as if she has shed a few years. Unlike the combined oral contraceptive (the pill), HRT medication does not usually contain synthetic hormones; it is mostly made from natural hormones derived from animal sources and contains smaller quantities of hormones than the pill that are designed to reproduce a woman's pre-menopausal hormonal levels. This means it can be taken safely by women for whom the pill was not suitable, either because it caused side effects or because they were already at an increased risk of thrombosis.

There are many forms of HRT, including skin patches, pills, creams and pessaries in varying combinations and doses of hormones, so if one type should prove unsuitable another might be more satisfactory. It may be necessary to go through a period of trial and error with different types of treatment to find the one that suits the individual woman best. A few women will not be able to use HRT for medical reasons and others prefer to avoid hormonal treatment altogether. In any case, if your symptoms are relatively minor or can be managed by other means, you may feel that you do not need it at all.

Many women are put off the whole idea of HRT because of scare stories in the media about associated health risks, but although possible risks do need to be considered carefully, many have been wildly exaggerated. These are summarized on page 43. When weighing up whether to begin HRT, you should obviously consider the possible benefits, both short- and long-term, as well as potential disadvantages for you personally, and your doctor or the staff at a menopause clinic should be able to provide you with all the information you need and give realistic advice. It is important that you are confident that taking HRT is the right course for you, otherwise you are less likely to stick with it once you have begun.

what is HRT?

As is clear from its name, the medication is designed to provide a substitute for those hormones that a woman's body produces in much reduced quantities from the menopause onwards. Prior to the cessation of her periods, as we have seen, levels will have been tailing off for some time, and they drop dramatically after the menopause, although small quantities of oestrogen are still secreted by fat cells and the adrenal glands. When HRT was first introduced in the last century, only oestrogen was given, until it was recognized that this treatment increased the risk of a woman developing cancer of the endometrium (the lining of the uterus). This problem was solved by adding progestogen (a synthetic form of progesterone) to protect the endometrium and this form of HRT is now prescribed for all women except those who have had their uterus surgically removed by a hysterectomy operation. Treatment may be prescribed on a short- or long-term basis, depending on circumstances and the woman's personal preference.

different types of HRT

In its earliest days, back in the 1930s, oestrogen was given first by injection and then by pellets but neither of these methods of administration is used today. All HRT is oestrogen-based because it is the lack of this hormone that is responsible for menopause-related symptoms; the treatment is given because post-menopausal women are regarded as being in an oestrogen-deficient state.

Most women take oestrogen in combination with progestogen to induce a regular bleed in which the uterine lining is shed as in a normal menstrual period. Although most oestrogens used in HRT are natural, synthetic rather than natural progesterone is used because in its natural form its effects are short-lived and unreliable. It is added to the oestrogen component either as tablets or in patches combined with oestrogen. Depending on the particular regime prescribed, progestogen may be taken for part or all of each treatment cycle (see page 40).

The hormones may be taken in a variety of forms and combinations, depending on the specific treatment being prescribed.

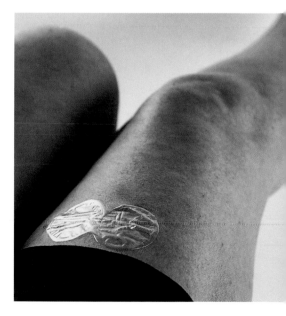

oestrogen	progestogen
Tablets	Tablets
Patches	Patches (together with oestrogen)
Implants	
Gels	
Creams	
Pessaries	
Vaginal rings	

There are various different ways of taking HRT and these different methods result in different bleeding patterns.

ABOVE: HRT patches are easy to use. They deliver a relatively low hormone dose, which produces fewer side-effects than tablets.

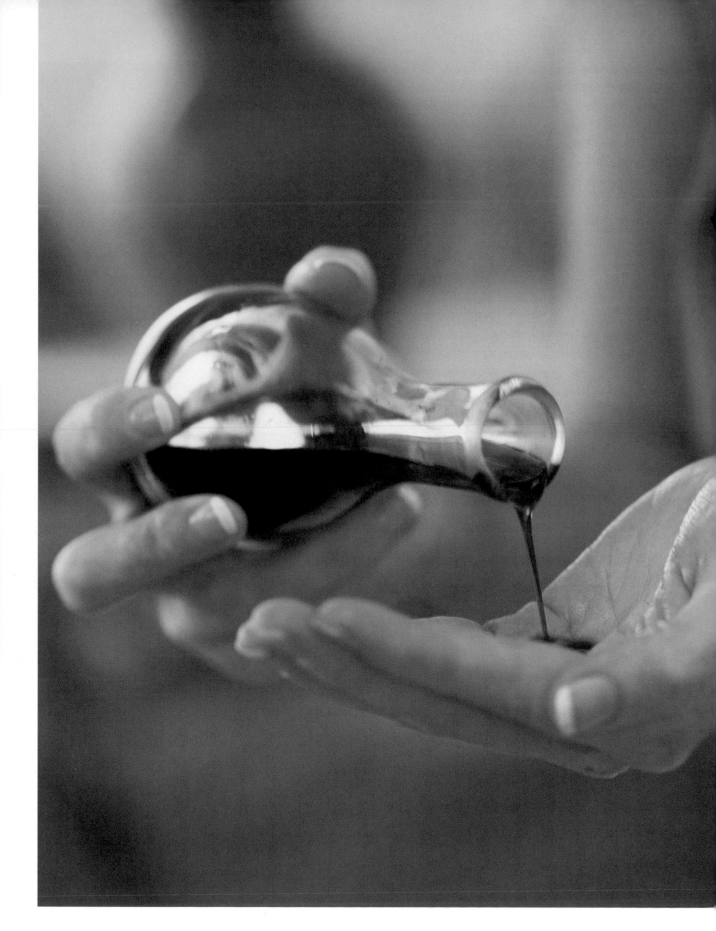

chapter 5

The growth in the popularity of complementary therapies over recent years has been phenomenal and the huge range of options can be confusing. Some, such as acupuncture and herbal medicine, have been used for centuries, while others, such as homoeopathy and Bach flower remedies, are of more recent origin. **Many people turn to complementary therapies for help with chronic conditions** that cannot be cured by orthodox medicine, while others use them to relieve stress or simply to enhance their overall sense of wellbeing. One of the main attractions of complementary medicine is that **it takes a holistic approach**; in other words, its practitioners aim to treat the whole person and not just the symptoms or the disease itself. Side effects are rare and generally minor, although more caution will be needed with powerful therapies such as herbal medicine. Before you consult a complementary therapist, it is wise to discuss your plans with your doctor in case the complementary therapy would not be appropriate or would conflict with the conventional treatment already being prescribed. However, in most cases your doctor is likely to give the go-ahead – conventionally trained doctors are becoming more open-minded about complementary therapies, even though some still adopt a sceptical approach.

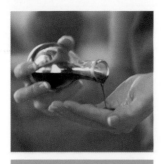

complementary
therapies

using complementary therapies

Generally, it is safe to use both complementary and conventional medicine at the same time. You should be wary of a complementary therapist who advises or encourages you to give up any existing conventional treatment and should not follow this advice without first consulting your doctor. Most therapists, however, will be happy to treat you in partnership with your doctor and will discuss any treatment you are currently receiving before treating you themselves. Many complementary therapies are suitable for self-treatment, but if at all possible it is best to consult a properly qualified practitioner, at least initially, to discuss how to go about treating yourself. Around the time of the menopause, many women find themselves having to deal with issues such as fear of ageing and life changes such as children leaving home or relationship difficulties at the same time as suffering troublesome physical symptoms. Many find that complementary therapy enables them to cope better with both emotional and physical problems and helps them to remain calm and to feel in control when life is difficult. Restoring natural balance is a big theme of many types of complementary therapies and this makes them especially appropriate around the time of the menopause, when hormonal imbalances are a major source of trouble. Different therapists will approach the task of rebalancing in different ways, but all will focus on the individual woman and her personal, unique needs when devising a treatment plan.

choosing a therapy

If you have never tried complementary therapy before, your best approach is to find out as much as you can about what's available and then simply start with the one that holds most appeal for you. You might want to consider whether you would prefer something relatively straightforward and practical, such as massage or osteopathy; or a more gentle treatment, such as aromatherapy or reflexology; or something with a more philosophical basis, such as yoga or acupuncture. Some people like the idea of remedies that can be seen as affecting the body directly, in which case homoeopathy, herbalism or Bach flower remedies would be a good choice.

If you are taking HRT or other medication you can continue to do so while having complementary treatment. Your therapist will ask you about current treatment, how you feel about it and whether it is effective. He or she will also want to know details of your general lifestyle, including your diet, work and sleep habits, emotional state and stress levels – in fact everything that might be contributing to your mental and physical health or lack of it. You should be prepared for a fairly lengthy question and

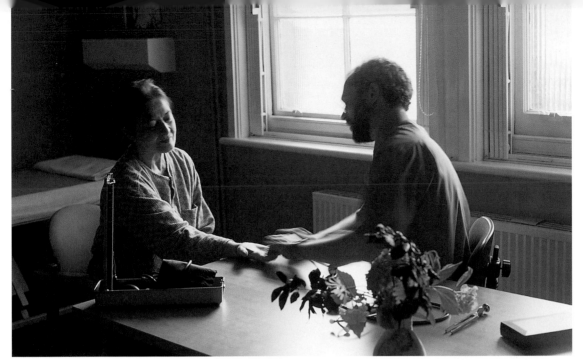

answer session before any treatment begins since it is essential for the therapist to know as much as possible about you before deciding on the appropriate course of treatment.

Your choice of therapies may be limited depending on where you live; in some countries legislation controls what therapies are permitted. In general, however, there is no requirement for therapists to belong to a recognized professional body, although the majority probably do so voluntarily. This means it is up to you to check out the therapist of your choice: ask about what type of training they have had, how long it lasted and what qualifications they have. If they do belong to a professional organization, you may also want to contact them for advice. You can also contact such organizations to find a list of therapists in your area. When making contact with a practitioner, ask them to give an indication of what they charge for a treatment session and if you can have an initial consultation before you make a final decision about whether to have treatment.

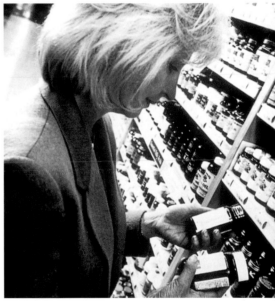

TOP: Before treatment begins, the therapist will ask many questions about you and your lifestyle to assess what treatment you need.

ABOVE: Some treatments, such as aromatherapy oils and Bach flower remedies, can be purchased for self-treatment, but it is always preferable to see a qualified practitioner first.

When you meet the practitioner and have discussed your health and possible treatment, ask how many sessions you can expect to need, how frequent they should be and how soon you can expect to see results. Use the initial consultation to assess whether you feel this particular therapist is someone with whom you could establish a rapport and, most importantly, whether you have confidence and trust in him or her. While what you say about yourself and the details of your treatment are confidential, you may find that you share personal information with your therapist which you would not confide to even your nearest and dearest, so it is important that you feel comfortable about the idea of doing this before you begin. No responsible therapist will promise anything approaching a miracle cure, whatever your symptoms, and you should distrust anyone who implies that this is a possibility.

natural therapies

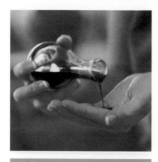

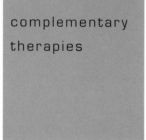

complementary
therapies

RIGHT: Aromatherapy oils can be used in many different ways that allow them to be either inhaled, as when used with a candle, or absorbed through the skin, as in massage.

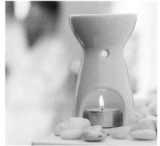 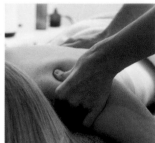

AROMATHERAPY

The word means 'treatment using scents' and refers to the use of essential oils derived from a variety of natural sources either individually or in combinations according to the needs of the person concerned. The oils are aromatic essences extracted from plants, flowers, trees, bark, grasses and seeds, each of which has its own distinctive therapeutic properties. They are very often used in combination with carrier oils for massage, but may also be added to bath water, inhalations, candles or skin sprays so that they are either absorbed through the skin or inhaled, or both.

Many oils have more than one therapeutic quality: among the most beneficial are their antiseptic properties; their digestive and diuretic effects; their power to promote relaxation and pain relief; and their anti-inflammatory, anti-viral and anti-depression effects. Practitioners believe that the oils work both in a direct physical way and through their influence on the mind and the emotions. When the therapist has chosen or blended the oils appropriate for your needs, you will be asked whether the aroma appeals to you. Be honest – a scent that you dislike is unlikely to have the desired effect. It is important that you give the therapist full details of any condition, current treatment or allergies. This will influence the choice of oils, as some may not be suitable if you have certain conditions, such as

raised blood pressure or epilepsy, for example. If you are opting to treat yourself, you should ideally consult a trained therapist first, but otherwise be sure to read the instructions, especially any warnings about conditions or medications that render a particular oil unsuitable for you. The other important cautionary note is that you must always check whether any essential oil you buy has already been diluted in carrier oil and, if it has not, do this yourself before applying it to your skin. You should never apply neat oil directly to your skin as it could cause an adverse reaction.

Essential oil of cypress is especially good for menopausal symptoms because it has cooling, drying qualities which help alleviate nervous tension, and a restful, woody smell. Use it in a burner or try adding it, together with a few drops each of clary sage, rosemary and lemon oils, to bath water. To make a cooling mist which will ease hot flushes, put 2 teaspoonfuls of cider vinegar into a spray bottle and top up with 100ml of still, bottled water, then add 3 drops each of cypress and clary sage essential oils, and shake before using.

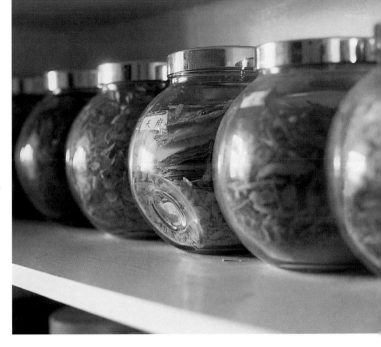

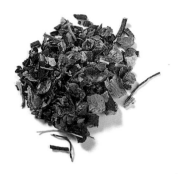

LEFT: Black cohosh is a North American herb used to restore hormone balance and reduce symptoms of the menopause.

RIGHT: There are many different herbs and the therapist will find a combination that suits you.

HERBAL MEDICINE

There are two different schools of herbal medicine which, though based on similar principles, use different methods of diagnosis and different preparations: Western and Chinese herbalism. Both approaches, however, use the whole herb, in contrast to orthodox medicines, which frequently use extracts from plants or synthetic analogues. As with homoeopathy, herbal remedies are designed to support the body and promote its natural healing abilities. Herbal medicines come in a variety of forms, including tinctures, creams, compresses, tablets and capsules, or as infusions such as teas and decoctions.

Chinese medicine has been used for over five thousand years and works on balancing the body's natural energy (called *chi*) and especially on equalizing the balance between the Yin and the Yang, which are often seen as female and male qualities. The practitioner will choose remedies designed to work on specific imbalances to restore the person to wholeness in body, mind and spirit. You should not try to treat yourself but always consult a qualified practitioner, because the herbs can have powerful effects and wrongly used can be toxic. Usually you will be given selected herbs to prepare as drinks at home – and the taste can take some getting used to!

Popular treatments include *Nuo dao gen* and *Wu wei zi* for night sweats, *Quing huo* and *My dan pi* for hot flushes, *Bao shao yao* and *Sang shen zi* for hair loss and *Du fu zi* and *Chi shao yao* for dry, itchy skin.

Western herbalists also use plant remedies to restore balance and promote good health through enhancing what they call the 'vital force'. Stress, poor diet and pollution can weaken this force and illness is the result of its efforts to maintain harmony when the body is under threat. The aim of treatment is not merely to fight illness but also to prevent recurrences, detoxify the body and support the immune system. St John's wort is a herbal remedy, long used to treat depression, which has recently been shown in scientifically controlled studies to be extremely effective and to have few side effects. A popular menopausal medicine is black cohosh, which is used to restore hormonal balance, thus helping to alleviate mood swings, depression, heavy bleeding and other symptoms related to oestrogen decline.

HOMOEOPATHY

This therapy, devised in the nineteenth century by Dr Samuel Hahnemann, works on the principle that 'like cures like'. In other words, a substance that triggers certain symptoms when taken can also cure the same symptoms when they result from disease or illness. There are over two thousand different remedies, derived from vegetable, mineral and animal sources and prepared by a process of multiple dilutions and shakings. Finally the liquid, which retains no measurable trace of the original substance, is added to inert pills, which are then prescribed on an individual basis. The remedies are designed to stimulate and support the body's own healing systems, which means that symptoms may get worse before they get better. It is possible to treat yourself, but a consultation with a qualified practitioner is likely to be more successful, as the remedies can then be tailored more specifically to your needs.

Lachesis, pulsatilla and amyl nit are among the most effective treatments for menopausal symptoms such as heavy bleeding, hot flushes and night sweats, and depression.

ACUPUNCTURE

Another element of traditional Chinese medicine, acupuncture is also based on the concept of restoring the free flow and balance of *chi*. This 'life force' is believed to flow along invisible channels in the body called meridians, and treatment is given by applying very fine needles to particular acupuncture points on the skin along the line of the meridians. Most people find the needles make the skin tingle but are not painful. It can be very helpful for symptoms such as migraine, hot flushes, heavy periods and poor skin tone, as well as for psychological problems such as poor memory and concentration.

RIGHT: Many Western doctors now prescribe acupuncture for their patients as this safe and painless treatment appears to have a good rate of success with many conditions.

BACH FLOWER REMEDIES

These are most appropriate for symptoms which are emotionally based. They were devised by Dr Bach with the aim of healing and eliminating the negative thoughts and feelings that can underlie both physical and mental symptoms. There are 38 different remedies, each tailored for a particular personality, attitude and state of mind, and they can be used individually or in combination. They can safely and effectively be used for home treatment and may enhance the benefits derived from other types of complementary therapy. Common menopausal remedies include walnut for life changes, mustard for unexplained depression, olive for fatigue, mimulus for fear of ageing, star of Bethlehem for sadness over lost youth and scleranthus for unexplained mood swings.

CHIROPRACTIC AND OSTEOPATHY

These are both types of manipulative therapy and are similar, although slightly different techniques are used and chiropractors may concentrate more on the spine and nervous system. They can be very helpful for people with joint or muscle problems and poor skeletal alignment, and can also help to relieve tension, which results in emotional as well as physical symptoms. Like other complementary therapists, practitioners take a holistic approach and the techniques are generally neither violent nor painful. However, these therapies must be used with caution for anyone with osteoporosis and joint conditions such as arthritis.

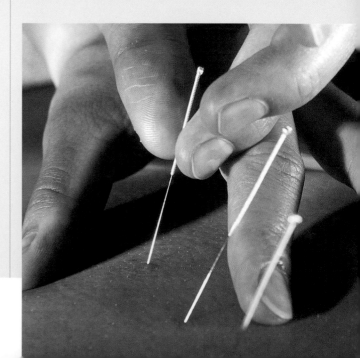

REFLEXOLOGY

A relatively modern form of treatment perfected during the last century, reflexology works by stimulating points on the feet or, sometimes, on the hands. Therapists visualize the feet and hands as a kind of mirror of the body, and every part of the body has its counterpoint on the feet and hands. The aim is to restore the proper balance of energy through the ten longitudinal zones which run from the extremities through the body to the head. By applying carefully placed pressure to the appropriate reflexes, therapists aim to improve overall physical and mental wellbeing, as well as to treat specific symptoms and conditions. Most people find the treatment sessions relaxing and enjoyable, and the practitioner may recommend simple methods of self-treatment to be used between sessions. Special attention is likely to be devoted to reflexes such as the pituitary, thyroid and adrenal glands to ease menopausal symptoms.

MASSAGE

Traditional massage can not only relieve muscular tension, joint pains and general aches and discomfort but also work wonders in relieving stress and emotional problems. There are many different schools of massage which differ in both their techniques and their underlying philosophy. Your choice will depend on what holds the most appeal for you personally, as well as what is on offer in your area. Traditional Swedish massage using oils on the skin is available almost everywhere and you may find other styles, such as Japanese shiatsu (or acupressure), Indian head massage or rolfing. Although you can learn simple techniques of self-massage, you really need to go to a qualified and experienced practitioner to gain the maximum benefits. Your therapist will need to know details of any existing health problems, such as arthritis or varicose veins, for example, as well as any menopausal symptoms, in order to treat you correctly. Mental and physical tension, headaches, bloating, period pains, mood swings, depression and irritability all respond well to massage and most people find the whole experience relaxing and uplifting.

HYDROTHERAPY

As water is an important constituent in our body's make-up, it should not surprise us that it can be used therapeutically. It is vital to keep properly hydrated, which means drinking around 2.5 litres of water every day; this doesn't include tea and coffee, which actually deplete your system of water because they have diuretic properties. If you are losing a lot of fluid as a result of hot flushes and night sweats, keeping up your water intake is even more important. Among its many functions in the body, water helps to keep the skin moist and supple, lubricates the joints, keeps the digestive and elimination system working properly and maintains the natural cooling system.

As well as taking in water as a drink, you can use it in various forms of therapy to help boost your circulation and promote the elimination of toxins. Showering or sitting in alternate hot and cold water is food for the circulation, although you should not use this technique if you have a heart condition. Even something as simple as a hot-water bottle or an ice pack can ease pain such as abdominal cramps and headaches.

NUTRITIONAL THERAPY

A nutritional therapist uses carefully selected diets to help promote optimum health, as well as to alleviate particular symptoms and conditions. You may believe that you already eat well, but a nutritional therapist will want to consider all aspects of your diet and lifestyle, together with any particular menopausal symptoms, before recommending changes to bring about health benefits. Despite the wide range of food available, many people in Western countries are overfed and undernourished at the same time, because they eat the wrong foods or have poor-quality diets. Some practitioners may use a range of techniques that they claim will diagnose allergies and food intolerance, sensitivity or deficiencies, but in general these are unreliable. Many allergies can be diagnosed by skin-patch or blood tests, but other methods are largely ineffective and usually inaccurate.

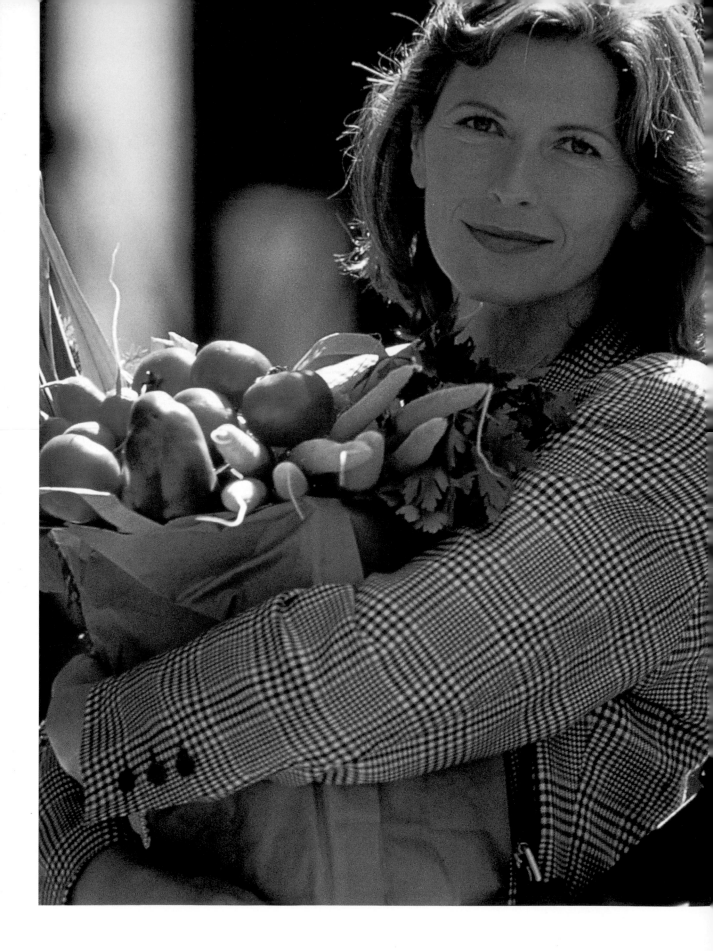

By choosing the right foods **you can boost your overall health and sense of wellbeing** and alleviate some of the symptoms of the menopause. Throughout life, a healthy, well-balanced diet is essential to maintain optimum functioning of all the systems in the body. As well as ensuring that you eat a **varied range of foods**, you should opt for natural foods whenever you can and keep processed and especially 'junk' food to an absolute minimum. If your diet is well balanced, it will provide you with all the vitamins and minerals you need.

Paying attention to your diet – **being aware of what you are eating and how your body responds to food** – is of the utmost importance. By adopting a healthy eating plan you will also help to maintain your weight at the right level for your height; this is an important consideration around the time of the menopause when women have a natural tendency to gain weight because of hormonal changes.

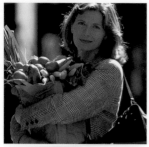

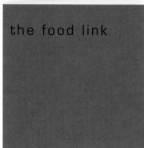

the food link

In the following pages, you will find the guidelines you need to ensure that your diet is as healthy as possible, but even if you already follow most of them, you will find suggestions as to some specific foods which have particular benefits as far as menopausal symptoms are concerned. If these are not already on your regular shopping list, it is worth adding them as they can play an important role in the production of natural oestrogen and help to regulate the hormonal fluctuations that occur at this time of bodily changes. You may find that they help to limit symptoms such as hot flushes, as well as improving your general physical and mental wellbeing during and after your menopause.

changing your diet

When thinking about any changes you plan to make in your eating habits, bear in mind that your aim is to improve your hormone balance and avoid anything that will increase the effects of changing levels on the way you feel. Three important factors to consider are:

the amounts and types of fats and fibre in your diet
foods which can contribute directly to levels of oestrogen and progesterone in your body
the benefits of specific nutrients

BELOW: Many beverages, including tea, coffee and alcohol, may prevent our bodies from getting all the nutrients they need.

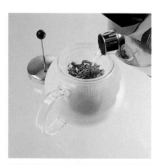

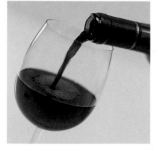

Our increased reliance on convenience and refined foods these days, together with the techniques of modern farming, have changed the quality of the food that most of us eat. Nutrients such as vitamins and minerals may be lost, wholly or partly, during refining and processing, and it is very easy to consume large amounts of substances which not only have no nutritional benefits but may even be counterproductive from a health point of view. For example, coffee, tea, cola drinks and alcohol all interfere with nutritional balance and may prevent you from obtaining all the essential nutrients your body needs to function properly. It goes without saying, of course, that smoking exacerbates the effects of a poor or unbalanced diet and again can prevent the proper absorption of vital nutrients such as vitamin C.

Drinking too much tea and coffee, eating too many sugary foods and snacks or having too many drinks that are high in sugar can result in fluctuating blood sugar levels, food cravings, headaches and fatigue. Cutting them back or changing to alternatives such as green tea, herbal teas, diluted fruit juice, fruit and yogurts will give you more energy and make you feel better.

making a plan

It is all too easy to become so confused about what you are going to eat that you give up all attempts to change your diet before you have started. The best way to proceed is to draw up a menu plan, which you can then use to make shopping lists. You could start by devising an overall programme of the changes you plan to make during the next three months and base your detailed eating plan on this. At the end of the three months, if you have managed to follow it fairly closely, you should already begin to notice changes in the way you feel. Any menopausal symptoms are likely to improve over this period and this will encourage you to stick with your new way of eating.

Think of your three-month programme as a guide to getting the best from the food that you eat, without too many dramatic changes to begin with. Simply developing an awareness of which foods are good for you and which should be reduced or avoided is a big step in the right direction. Use the list below as a kind of route map and this will make it easier to work your way through the detailed recommendations that follow.

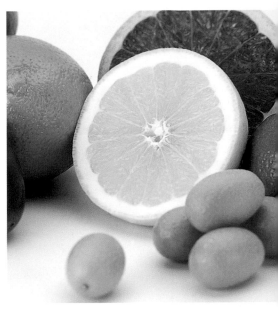

ABOVE: Fresh fruits are packed with vitamins.

basic principles

→ **Drink six to eight glasses of water a day**, preferably bottled or filtered.

→ **Eat at least five servings of fresh fruit and vegetables daily**, raw or lightly cooked and organic if possible, to boost your vitamin and mineral intake.

→ **Reduce your intake of refined foods** – sweets, cakes, biscuits, sugar, junk food, jam, puddings, chocolate and sugary drinks. Many people think of honey as being a naturally healthy food but although it may contain tiny quantities of minerals, it is really just another form of sugar with little in the way of nutrients.

→ **Choose low-fat dairy products** and remember that you can also boost your calcium intake by eating more sardines, broccoli, salmon, lentils and nuts.

→ **Reduce your overall fat intake**. Calories from fat should comprise no more than a third of your overall daily consumption. Be especially wary of 'hidden' fat in foods such as ready-made meals, crisps, pies and sausages and cut down on ordinary margarine and oils. Any fat which is solid at room temperature – for example, lard – is likely to be saturated fat; the same holds true for fat from animal sources, which includes butter and also the visible fat on meat, so choose lean meat or remove all visible fat before cooking. Limit red meat to one or two portions a week. Try fish, poultry, pulses, nuts and rice (preferably brown) instead.

→ **The body does need some fat** but the best types are polyunsaturated (oils such as corn oil, safflower, sunflower and soya bean oil) and monounsaturated (olive oil). Virgin cold-pressed olive oil tastes good and is ideal for cooking and salad dressings.

→ **Change to herb teas, green tea and dandelion coffee** and cut back on ordinary tea and coffee, which contain the stimulant caffeine.

→ **Alcohol does you no harm in moderation** and there is some evidence that a daily glass of wine may actually be good for you, but it is important not to overdo your consumption. Limit yourself to 3 units per day.

→ **Limit your salt intake** and be aware of 'hidden' salt in foods such as packet soup, cereals and pickles.

optimum nutrition

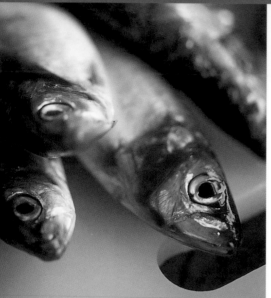

Many nutritionists and dieticians, as well as food scientists, now talk of 'nutriceuticals', which can be translated as meaning foods that have positive therapeutic and medicinal effects. The familiar expression 'you are what you eat' is true in the general sense that your health and wellbeing depend to a very great extent on what you put into your body.

While modern intensive farming methods and the availability of foods from all parts of the world, regardless of the season, have given us more choice than in any previous era, the production methods used, including hormones, fertilizers and pesticides, and the gap between harvesting or producing the food and its consumption may reduce its nutritional value. Nevertheless, by taking care when planning menus, you can ensure your meals are healthy and well balanced, as well as being enjoyable.

To make healthy eating easier, it is useful to take account of the various food 'groups' which need to be included in your diet. These are carbohydrates, proteins, fruit and vegetables, fats, vitamins and minerals, and together they comprise the basic components of a nutritious and balanced diet.

CARBOHYDRATES

Most nutritionists agree that carbohydrates should provide around 60 per cent of daily calories, but the picture is slightly complicated by the fact that they come in two forms. The more desirable are complex carbohydrates, such as root vegetables, cereals, rice, pulses and legumes, pasta and some fruits. It is better to opt for the unrefined forms – whole-meal bread, rice, pasta and breakfast cereals, for example – because much of the nutritional content is lost when these foods are refined into their 'white' form. The unrefined versions are also broken down more slowly in the gut, which means they release energy (glucose) into the bloodstream at a slow rate. This is not the case with simple carbohydrates, such as sugar, which produce a rapid rise in blood glucose levels, stimulating the release of insulin from the pancreas, which causes blood glucose to fall with equal rapidity.

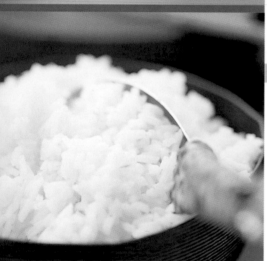

TOP: Oily fish such as sardines contain protein as well as many other beneficial nutrients.

ABOVE: Rice is a good source of carbohydrate.

PROTEINS

These are often called the body's building blocks, but you need fewer of them than you might think. They should provide no more than 15 per cent of your daily calorie consumption. All the main organs of the body are created from protein; skin, bone, muscle tissue and hair all contain protein and they are important for the effective functioning of the immune system. When you eat large amounts of protein, the body stores the excess in muscles and organs. Protein is broken down into amino acids by enzymes during digestion and these are absorbed into the bloodstream and used to repair tissue and muscles. Good sources include meat, fish, poultry, nuts, dairy produce and pulses.

FRUIT AND VEGETABLES

These are absolutely vital to maintain good health and contain many natural chemicals which help to protect against a wide range of illnesses. You should eat at least five portions a day (not counting potatoes) to ensure that you meet your body's vitamin requirements; the more you consume, the less likely you are to need vitamin supplements. Of particular importance are the antioxidant vitamins and minerals, vitamins C, E, beta-carotene (which is converted into vitamin A in the body) and selenium, a trace mineral found in the soil. These are known to promote good health and protect from disease by aiding the body's natural defences against damage by free radicals – chemicals produced naturally in the body which limit the effectiveness of the immune system. The so-called 'ACE' vitamins are provided by dark, leafy vegetables such as broccoli and spinach and yellow-orange fruits and vegetables such as apricots, mangoes, carrots, sweet potatoes, red peppers, citrus fruits and avocados.

All fruit and vegetables should be thoroughly washed before cooking or eating raw to remove any chemicals on the skin, although if you opt for organically grown produce this should not be a problem.

antioxidants

Antioxidants (vitamins C, E and beta-carotene, a precursor of vitamin A) help to control the unstable molecules called free radicals that, when produced in excess, can attack and damage various cells in the body. Sunlight, smoking, illness, pollution and stress can trigger over-production of free radicals. As well as damaging the cellular structure of arteries and other tissue, they may affect collagen – the scaffolding which supports the skin – so that it starts to look leathery and tough, creating wrinkles, creases and bags under the eyes. Antioxidants are believed to slow down the damage caused by free radicals and are present in minerals such as selenium, zinc, manganese and iron, as well as in the 'ACE' vitamins. Green tea is a good source of antioxidants and is a refreshing drink first thing in the morning, especially if you are trying to cut down on your consumption of ordinary tea and coffee.

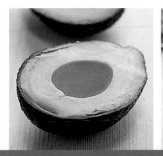
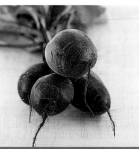

LEFT: All fresh fruits and vegetables are beneficial in the diet, and it is important, and more enjoyable, to include as wide a range as possible. Avocados are especially full of vitamins and minerals.

nutrients essential for good skin

NUTRIENT	WHAT IT DOES	WHERE TO FIND IT	PROTECTS AGAINST
Vitamin A	Antioxidant; helps to slow down the accumulation of keratin and keep the skin supple	Oily fish; offal; eggs; dairy foods; orange and yellow fruits, including peaches	Scaly skin; flaky scalp; acne; poor wound healing
Beta-carotene (pro-vitamin A)	Provides the body with the components to manufacture vitamin A; protects against the ageing effects of ultraviolet light and boosts immunity	Carrots; dark green vegetables; apricots; oranges; tomatoes; peppers; sweet potatoes; squash; pumpkin; watercress; cabbage; broccoli	As for vitamin A
Bioflavonoids	Antioxidant; slows down the deterioration of connective tissue and strengthens the small capillaries that feed the skin. Strengthens capillaries, preserves collagen, protects against osteoporosis, strengthens walls of vagina, promotes healthy cell structures	Pith and segments of citrus fruits; apricots; blackberries; cherries; rose hips; apples; buckwheat	Easy bruising; slow wound healing; premature ageing
Vitamin B2	Necessary for the development and repair of healthy skin tissue	Milk; eggs; cereals; liver; green leafy vegetables; mackerel; mushrooms	Seborrhoeic dermatitis or inflammation around the nose and mouth; cracked lips; dull or oily hair
Vitamin B3	Helps the skin produce natural sunscreening substances, such as melanin	Brown rice; chicken; wheatgerm; tuna; broccoli	Dermatitis; acne; eczema; fatigue; depression
Vitamin B5 (panthothenic acid)	Necessary for the formation of new skin tissue to maintain healthy hair	Yeast; liver; kidney; eggs; brown rice; wholegrain cereals; lentils; wholemeal bread; nuts; dried fruits	Muscle tremors; cramps; fatigue; anxiety
Vitamin B6	Helps maintain normal oil balance in the skin and prevent allergic reactions; helps immune and nervous system	Chicken; yeast extract; broccoli; bananas; wheatgerm; beef; fish; eggs; brown rice; nuts; soya beans; whole grains	Overactive sebaceous glands, resulting in oily skin; flaky skin; water retention
Vitamin B12	Helps the blood carry oxygen to the skin; helps eliminate toxins	Red meat; liver; eggs; fish	Dry skin; dermatitis; pale complexion
Biotin	Helps the body use essential fats; moderates the output of overactive sebaceous glands	Offal; wheatgerm; brewer's yeast	Dry skin; eczema; scaly dermatitis
Vitamin C	Antioxidant, so helps protect against free radicals; helps manufacture collagen; anti-bacterial, so helps to reduce infection on the skin; detoxifies, helping to eliminate waste; vital for production of collagen	most fruit and vegetables: blackcurrants; oranges; peppers; cherries; strawberries; broccoli; watercress	Broken thread veins; rough, scaly skin; easy bruising; red pimples; dry scalp

NUTRIENT	WHAT IT DOES	WHERE TO FIND IT	PROTECTS AGAINST
Vitamin E (tocopherol)	Helps prevent cell damage; strengthens blood vessels; maintains good circulation; antioxidant which helps to protect against oxidation of polyunsaturated fat cells in cell membranes; especially important if diet is rich in fish and polyunsaturated fats	Seeds; nuts; oily fish; sunflower oil; avocado; beans; wheatgerm	Premature wrinkles; pale skin; acne; easy bruising; slow wound healing
Folic acid	Slows down the loss of moisture from the skin	Brewer's yeast; liver; wheatgerm; molasses; green leafy vegetables; eggs; nuts; wholegrains	Dry skin; eczema; cracked lips; pale complexion
Calcium	Helps skin regeneration; maintains good acid-alkaline balance; helps prevent osteoporosis, essential for strong bones	Milk; cheese; yogurt; almonds; parsley; brewer's yeast; sesame seeds; kale; seaweed; turnips; almonds; soya beans; dandelion leaves; hazelnuts; honey; horseradish; salmon; dairy products	Sallow, 'tired' skin
Magnesium	Works with calcium to build and slow down the age-related shrinkage that produces wrinkles; essential for muscle activity; aids absorption of calcium to produce strong bones, needed to help prevent osteoporosis	Fresh green vegetables; raw wheatgerm; soya beans; milk; wholegrains; seafood; figs; apples; oily fish; nuts	Constipation, producing sallow and blemished skin; bone shrinkage; lack of energy
Selenium	Antioxidant, so fights free radicals; helps body use vitamin E; reduces inflammation	Herrings; molasses; tuna; oysters; mushrooms; wheatgerm; bran; onions; broccoli; shellfish	Dull complexion; dry skin
Silica	Needed for collagen manufacture	Horsetail (herb)	Premature wrinkles; eczema; psoriasis; acne; poor wound healing
Sulphur	FIghts bacterial infection to help keep skin clear; aids detoxification by stimulating bile secretion	Lean beef; dried beans; fish; eggs; cabbage	Dull complexion; skin infections; fatigue
Co-enzyme Q10	Supports immune system, so fights bacterial infection; antioxidant, so slows ageing caused by free radicals	Soya oils; sardines; mackerel; peanuts; pork	Depressed immunity; sallow skin
Zinc	Antioxidant; helps to make the protein that carries vitamin A to the skin; slows down the age-related weakening of collagen and elastin fibres; supports the immune system in destroying bacteria; helps strengthen bones	Meat; wholegrains; brewer's yeast; wheatbran; wheatgerm; soy lecithin; beans; apricots; peaches; oysters; mustard seeds; cocoa; pumpkin seeds; nectarines; eggs	Dull complexion; eczema; acne; limp, dull hair; white marks on fingernails

essential vitamins and minerals

NUTRIENT	FOOD SOURCES	BENEFITS
Vitamin A	Liver; eggs; carrots; spinach; broccoli; fruit	Eyesight; skin; possible protection against cancer
Vitamin C	Peppers; oranges; strawberries; blackcurrants	Helps heal wounds; may fight colds, flu and infections; protects gums; keeps joints and ligaments in good working order; antioxidant
Vitamin D	Tuna; salmon; mackerel; sardines; fish-liver oils; egg yolks	Aids absorption of calcium and phosphorus for healthy bones and teeth
Vitamin E	Green leafy vegetables; corn; avocado; asparagus; wheatgerm; wholegrain cereals; brown rice; pure vegetable oils; nuts; seeds; soya beans; tofu	Cell growth; antioxidant
Vitamin B1	Most foods including wheatgerm; wholegrain cereals; pulses; nuts	Helps the breakdown of carbohydrates; nervous system
Vitamin B2	Liver; kidney; dairy produce; eggs; brewer's yeast; wheat bran; wheatgerm	Repairs body tissue
Vitamin B3	Fish; wheatgerm; wholegrain cereals	Essential for chemical reactions
Vitamin B6	Lean meat; liver; fish; wholegrains; bananas; avocados; potatoes	Nervous system; skin; red blood cells
Vitamin B12	Liver; kidney; some fish; shellfish; eggs; milk	Blood and nerves
Vitamin K	Most vegetables, especially dark green leafy ones; liver	Helps in the production of some proteins
Calcium	Red meat; liver; oily fish; wholegrain cereals; leafy green vegetables	Bones, teeth and nails; muscles and nerve function
Copper	Turnips; peaches; shellfish; nuts; lentils	Helps prevent osteoporosis; antioxidant
Iron	Lean red meat; liver; pulses; dark green leafy vegetables; dried fruit	Makes haemoglobin, the pigment in red blood cells that helps transport oxygen around the body
Magnesium	Lean meat; fish; shellfish; pulses; brown rice; green vegetables; bananas; nuts; seeds	Regulates thyroid hormones and protects against artery clogging; cancels out the pollutants in the body
Potassium	Bananas; citrus fruits; dried fruits; nuts; seeds; potatoes; pulses	Keeps up energy levels – releases energy from the muscles; stops blood sugar fluctuations which can cause dizziness and tiredness; needed for production of cells, bone, proteins and fatty acids
Selenium	Lean meat; liver; fish; shellfish; brazil nuts; wholegrain cereals; tomatoes; broccoli; onions	Maintains normal blood pressure and regular heartbeat; facilitates transmission of nerve impulses
Zinc	Red meat; sardines; shellfish; root vegetables; nuts; seeds	Boosts immune system; improves red blood cells

Fats are an essential part of a healthy diet but you need to know which ones are beneficial to health and which ones are not. Most foods contain varying amounts of saturated, polyunsaturated and monounsaturated fats.

Saturated fats – derived mainly from animal sources, these are found in such foods as meat, butter, full-fat milk, lard and cheese, as well as coconut oil, margarine and processed meat products such as sausages, salami, burgers, pâté and bacon. They contribute to obesity because of their high calorie content and can also increase blood cholesterol levels and encourage the development of atheroma, which can clog up arteries.

Trans-fatty acids – these fats are found in many hard margarines and spreads, as well as in processed foods such as pies, crisps, biscuits, cakes and some meat and dairy products. There have been suggestions that trans-fatty acids might be harmful because they trigger the production of free radicals – molecules that can damage cell structure. They are also linked to obesity, furring of the arteries and high levels of cholesterol.

Polyunsaturated fats – these are found in oily fish, nuts, seeds and some vegetables. There are two basic types, omega-6 (linoleic acid) and omega-3 (linolenic acid), both of which perform several essential roles within the body. Omega-6 EFAs (essential fatty acids) are found in nuts, seeds and vegetable oils, especially corn, safflower, soya, sunflower and walnut oils. Omega-3 EFAs are present in oily fish, such as mackerel, herrings and sardines, and in walnuts and rapeseed oil. These oils are particularly important in keeping skin from becoming dry and they help to maintain a healthy metabolism and good joint mobility. They contribute to preventing heart disease – an increased risk for post-menopausal women – by reducing the blood's tendency to clot. They also play a vital part in maintaining a healthy nervous system and immune system and promote good fluid balance in the body, which may help with symptoms such as fluid retention. Linseed (flax) oil is a particularly rich source of EFAs and contains beta-carotene and vitamin E. It is not suitable for cooking but can be added to salads or mixed with other foods, especially yogurt.

Monounsaturated fats – sometimes known as omega-9, are a useful substitute for saturated fats and some also contain EFAs. Olive oil is the best known, but other sources include avocados, nuts, seeds and rapeseed oil. The relatively low rates of cardiovascular disease in some Mediterranean countries have been ascribed in part to high consumption of olive oil, although it is likely that other factors are also relevant.

fibre

Fibre is a natural component of all plant-derived foods and comes from the cell walls. Although it has no nutritional value, it is essential for efficient digestion and elimination of waste products. It is important because it absorbs water from the digestive tract, making stools bulkier so they pass out through the body more smoothly and comfortably. Increasing the amount of fibre in your diet will also mean that glucose from the food you have eaten will be released into your bloodstream gradually rather than in a rush. There are two types of fibre: soluble – from fruit, vegetables, pulse and oats, for example; and insoluble – unrefined rice, nuts, fruit peel and bran. Some foods contain both types. Another advantage for those trying to control their weight is that a high-fibre diet helps you to feel full. In the past, bran was promoted as a good source of fibre, but because it is a refined food it can interfere with the effective absorption of nutrients such as zinc, magnesium and calcium. For this reason it is better to get your fibre from wholegrains, fruit, pulses and legumes, and vegetables. If your diet has previously been low in fibre, you should increase the amount you eat gradually to avoid 'wind' and indigestion, and make sure you drink plenty of water. Good sources of fibre include:

→ cooked and raw fresh fruit and vegetables
→ wholegrains such as brown rice, wholegrain crackers, wholemeal bread, wholemeal pasta, beans, nuts and seeds
→ muesli – try soaking it overnight to make it easier for your system to absorb the necessary nutrients

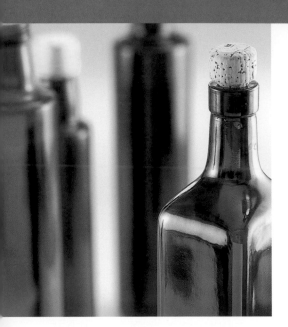

choosing and storing oils

When choosing oils, opt for the very best quality you can afford, as they will be the purest and least processed and thus offer more potential health benefits. Extra virgin olive oil, which is generally unrefined, and cold-pressed organic unrefined oils are the best choices. Unrefined oil is extracted without the use of heat, unlike sunflower oil, for example, and heat affects the quality and nutritional content, thus lowering the potential health benefits. You need to think about where you keep your oil, because it can be attacked by free radicals which causes oxidation. Store, preferably in dark rather than clear bottles, away from heat and sunlight, and don't overheat it when cooking.

ABOVE: Store oils in dark bottles in a cool dark place to prevent them oxidizing.

fat sense

For all their bad reputation as promoters of weight gain, as we have seen, fats are an essential component of our diet. The secret is to choose them carefully and then use them sparingly.

don't:

→ heat oils to too high a temperature

→ roast nuts – it destroys the nutrients in the oils

→ use hydrogenated margarine or those made with polyunsaturated vegetable oils that have been hydrogenated

→ store oils in the light, for example in clear bottles on the windowsill

Spread butter thinly or replace with unsaturated spread
Choose semi-skimmed or skimmed rather than full-fat milk
Trim off excess fat on meat and use leans cut whenever possible
Cook with liquid fats, preferably virgin olive oil, and use sparingly as salad dressings
Read food labels carefully – saturated fats are in many products, particularly refined and processed foods
Avoid or minimize your consumption of hidden saturated fats in cakes, biscuits and pastries
Grill rather than fry food
Regularly replace meat with fish, lentils and nuts

phytoestrogens

Phytoestrogens are plant foods that produce natural oestrogens and are similar in structure to the female hormone (the word *phyto* is Greek and means plant). They have about 1 per cent of the potency of our own oestrogen and can raise or lower oestrogen levels in the female body. In comparison with HRT they provide much less oestrogen, but they may nevertheless help to counteract the fall in levels that occurs at the time of the menopause. Phytoestrogens may also help to protect against heart disease and osteoporosis and are therefore important at this stage in a woman's life.

Most fruit, cereals and vegetables contain phytoestrogen in varying strengths. Those containing isoflavones are the most beneficial. These are found in legumes such as soya, chickpeas and lentils.

Until recently, it was believed that the high soya content of the Japanese diet was the reason why women in that country appeared to have fewer menopausal symptoms and less breast cancer than women who follow a Western diet. However, new research has questioned this assumption and it is now thought that the high fish intake in Japan might be the reason, though some soya consumption may still offer health benefits.

THE BENEFITS OF PHYTOESTROGENS

Research on the effects of soya has suggested that it may help to reduce hot flushes and night sweats, as well as reducing vaginal dryness and irritation. Soya beans have been found to contain at least five compounds believed to inhibit cancer, one of which is chemically similar to the drug tamoxifen, prescribed for women who have had oestrogen-dependent breast cancer to prevent a recurrence. The phytoestrogens and tamoxifen are believed to work in a similar way: that is, locking on to the oestrogen receptors and thus inhibiting cancer growth. Research is currently being undertaken to find out whether increasing the intake of phytoestrogens and isoflavones helps protect against breast cancer and osteoporosis. Some studies have indicated that soya may help to activate bone growth and therefore improve bone density, but further work is needed to establish whether it can play a role in preventing osteoporosis.

Phytoestrogens are also linked to the reduction of cholesterol in the body. Cholesterol is a blood fat that is found in all body tissues and is a constituent of atheroma, the fatty substance that can clog up arteries. The amount of cholesterol in your blood depends upon many factors, such as your age, diet, sex and lifestyle, but most importantly on your genetic

sources of phytoestrogens and isoflavones

→ **fruits** – apples, bananas, cherries, citrus fruits, cranberries, dates, figs, papaya, pomegranates, plums, rhubarb

→ **grains** – barley, oats, rice, rye, wheat

→ **herbs and spices** – fennel, parsley, red clover, sage and cinnamon

→ **pulses and legumes** – aduki beans, chickpeas, kidney beans, lentils, peas

→ **seaweed** – kelp, kombu, nori, wakame

→ **seeds** – caraway, linseed, pumpkin, poppy, sunflower

→ **soya and soya products** – miso (fermented soya beans used as flavouring for soups and casseroles), soya milk, tofu, soya flour

→ **sprouts** – alfalfa, mung beans

→ **vegetables** – beetroot, broccoli, carrots, celery, fennel, garlic, green beans, potatoes, yam

BELOW: Garlic and wheat, found in most types of bread, are good sources of phytoestrogens.

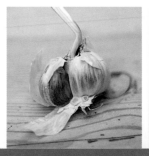
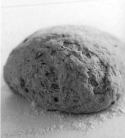

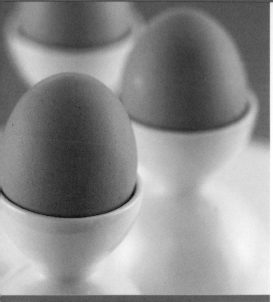

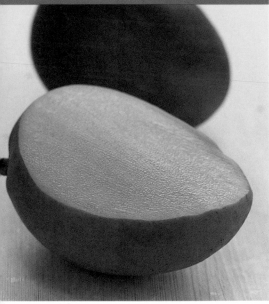

ABOVE: Eggs and mangoes are among the foods that are rich in minerals, which can be depleted by prolonged stress.

inheritance. There are two main forms: high-density lipid (HDL) and low-density lipid (LDL). The former is carried in the bloodstream to the liver for breakdown, while the latter is taken to the organs and tissues for use. LDL is the type that may stick to artery walls and impede blood flow. Before the menopause women usually have higher levels of HDL in their bloodstream and low levels of LDL, but after the menopause balance alters, increasing the risk of heart disease. Raising oestrogen levels can help reduce the risk significantly because it shifts the cholesterol balance in favour of HDL.

Although heredity is the most important factor in determining cholesterol levels, eating saturated fats can raise the level of LDL and foods containing phytoestrogens may help to lower them.

stress-busting foods

The adrenal glands that sit above the kidneys have many functions. They manufacture 28 individual hormones, help with the digestion of food, regulate the thyroid gland, top up energy levels and help the body to deal with stress. They also produce small amounts of oestrogen, which becomes more important after the menopause when ovarian production stops. Stress causes the body to use up its resources of minerals and vitamins rapidly. When you are in a situation that triggers stress, the adrenals release adrenaline and noradrenaline – the so-called stress hormones – to prepare you for tackling the 'danger' by flight or flight. As the situation is resolved, the adrenals return to normal, but if it is not resolved, production of stress hormones continues. In the long term, raised levels of stress hormones may interfere with the effective function of the immune system and leave you feeling tired, weak and sometimes completely fatigued.

Stress seems to be an inevitable part of life for most people today, whether it's mental or physical, and poor nutrition exacerbates its effects. Eating well will help your adrenal glands to function properly and your body to cope with the strains placed upon it by stressful situations and lifestyles. A good intake of vitamins and minerals is particularly important around the menopause as the body adapts to the hormonal changes taking place. Prolonged stress may deplete your body of important minerals such as magnesium, zinc, calcium, sodium, potassium and copper. Keep up your levels by eating a mineral-rich diet, including dark green vegetables, yellow-orange vegetables and fruit, legumes, pulses, wholegrains, eggs and meat.

sodium

The body needs sodium, but high levels of this mineral can be associated with raised blood pressure and affect the body's ability to balance fluid retention. Sodium chloride (common salt) is a major source of sodium in our bodies and the average Western diet contains large amounts; most people probably consume ten times more salt than they need. Many foods, such as fruit, vegetables and grains, already contain sodium, so adding salt to the diet to provide sodium is unnecessary.

Convenience and refined foods contain more salt than most people realize: burgers, biscuits, pizza, ketchup and salad dressings are just some of the culprits. By cutting down on processed foods and opting for fresh food instead, you can decrease your salt intake significantly. Avoid adding salt when cooking vegetables, for example, do not put extra on your food at the table and develop the habit of checking food labels for salt content.

controlling weight and mood swings

Maintaining a healthy weight is important at any age but especially during and after the menopause, when there is a natural tendency to put on extra kilos. Keeping active and taking regular exercise will counteract this. Excess weight can lead to many complications and can also increase the risk of heart disease and diabetes.

However, a small increase in weight during the menopause is acceptable because it helps to prevent oestrogen levels from falling too far. As the ovaries stop production, so the body fat acts as a supplementary source of oestrogen. Eating a healthy diet will keep your weight within acceptable limits and you may even find you lose a little. The food we consume is converted into energy or fat, and by eating the right types of food we can encourage out bodies to use it rather than store it as fat. The best types of food for energy are the complex carbohydrates, because as well as supplying energy they also keep blood sugars steady, which will help to prevent mood swings. To lose weight you have to consume less energy than you expend and changing your eating habits for good is always going to be preferable to going on crash diets. The latter can provide only a temporary solution, because after an initial loss you are virtually certain to put it back on again once you resume your old eating habits.

seaweed

Sometimes known as sea vegetable, seaweed is very low in calories and has a high mineral content, containing zinc, chromium, selenium, manganese, magnesium, calcium, iron and iodine. The latter is very important in helping to maintain a healthy thyroid gland, which regulates the metabolism. As the metabolic rate slows after the menopause, seaweed can be a useful addition to your diet; use it to flavour stews and soups. Many varieties are available in health food shops, including:

→ **agar** – sold in flake form; very high in fibre

→ **hijiki** – looks like tangled black string and tastes like liquorice; half a cup of cooked hijiki contains as much calcium as half a cup of milk

→ **kombu** – kelp, with a sweet/salty taste; high in magnesium, potassium, calcium, iron and iodine; can be toasted for snacks or sprinkled on other dishes

→ **nori** – sea lettuce, nutty-tasting and high in vitamins A and B; comes in sheets and you can wrap other food, such as rice, in it

→ **wakame** – a dark green leaf, it is a rich source of vitamins A, B complex and E

Also look out for dulse and arame.

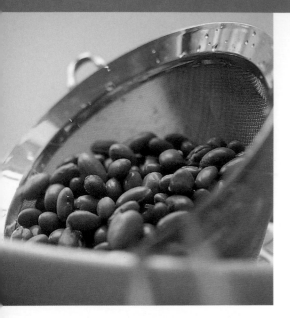

ABOVE: Beans provide plenty of essential fibre.

food allergies and intolerance

Adverse reactions to certain foods seem to be increasingly common, but it is important to distinguish between the various types. If you are allergic to particular foods, your body will react to them as if they were an alien invader such as a bacterium or virus. The immune system produces antibodies to fight off the invasion and in extreme cases this can result in a potentially fatal reaction known as anaphylactic shock. More commonly, however, an allergy results in symptoms such as skin rashes or eruptions, nausea and vomiting, and diarrhoea. People who are intolerant to a particular food usually have a reaction because their body lacks the ability to digest it properly; the most common examples are lactose intolerance (inability to digest milk protein) and coeliac disease (inability to digest gluten, a protein in wheat). Such conditions arise because the person lacks the digestive enzyme needed to process something in the particular food and symptoms may include serious digestive problems.

Food sensitivity is much more common and though unpleasant is not life-threatening. Symptoms may be vague but can include bloating, water retention, aching joints, digestive and skin problems, asthma, hyperactivity and migraine headaches. Often it turns out that the problem food is one you tend to crave. Cutting out suspect foods for a period may help identify the culprit(s), though this can be a difficult and time-consuming process. Stop eating all the foods you think may be troubling you for about three weeks, then reintroduce them one by one to see which causes a reaction. When you first cut them out you may find that you feel worse as you suffer withdrawal symptoms. If you add a food and it produces the reaction, take it back out again and wait until you stabilize before reintroducing another food. A qualified nutritionist can help devise a suitable programme for you to follow.

poor eating habits

Irregular meals, missing meals and low blood glucose levels can affect not only your health but also your moods. Eating little and often helps to stabilize blood glucose and it is important not to miss breakfast as blood glucose falls overnight. Complex carbohydrates are the ideal foods to keep blood glucose levels stable as they release energy slowly into the bloodstream. A banana or a slice of wholemeal toast is a good choice.

tips for healthy weight loss

→ Eat plenty of fresh fruit and vegetables, which are high in vitamins and low in calories
→ Increase fibre-rich foods such as fruit, vegetables, whole grains, beans and lentils
→ Eat more fish, poultry and lean meat
→ Avoid fried food
→ Cut down on fatty meat products such as sausages, pork pies and sausage rolls
→ Reserve cakes and pastries for special occasions
→ Choose low-fat dairy options
→ Drink plenty of water
→ Try to cut back on stimulants such as coffee and tea
→ Avoid alcoholic drinks – they are high in calories
→ Enjoy your food

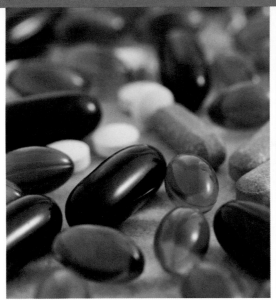

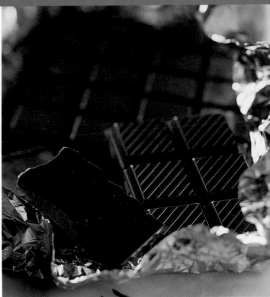

RIGHT: There is an overwhelming selection of vitamin and mineral supplements available. Ask your doctor to refer you to a dietician for reliable advice.

FAR RIGHT: Chocolate is one of the most common culprits in food allergies and intolerances.

Water is essential to maintain optimum health because it keeps the body properly hydrated; by the time you start to feel thirsty you are already dehydrated. Water flushes toxins from the body, stopping it becoming sluggish, cleans the system and repairs the cells. It helps to keep skin looking and feeling good from the inside out. Filtered or bottled mineral water is best and certain varieties contain trace minerals that are important for maintaining health.

supplements

Making the time to shop and prepare meals from scratch is not always easy, which is why we sometimes resort to convenience foods and take-aways. The danger there is that poor eating habits can result in a deficiency in essential nutrients. A massive industry has grown up to provide supplements, but the choice on offer in supermarkets, pharmacies and health food shops is vast and often confusing.

If you suspect you should be taking supplements, it is worth asking your doctor to refer you to a qualified dietician for expert advice. In particular, you should be wary of any products that claim to treat or cure specific conditions or serious symptoms. Ideally, you should not need to take supplements if you are eating a healthy, balanced and varied diet, and nutrients absorbed in their natural form from good food are far more beneficial than synthetic substitutes.

common culprit foods in allergies and intolerances

→ alcohol
→ chocolate
→ citrus fruits
→ coffee and caffeinated drinks such as chocolate, cocoa, cola and tea
→ dairy products
→ honey
→ peanuts
→ pickles and pickled products
→ processed and smoked meats, including bacon, frankfurters and salami
→ shellfish
→ smoked fish
→ spices and flavour enhancers such as monosodium glutamate (MSG)
→ strawberries
→ wheat and wheat products, including bread, cereals and pasta
→ yeast

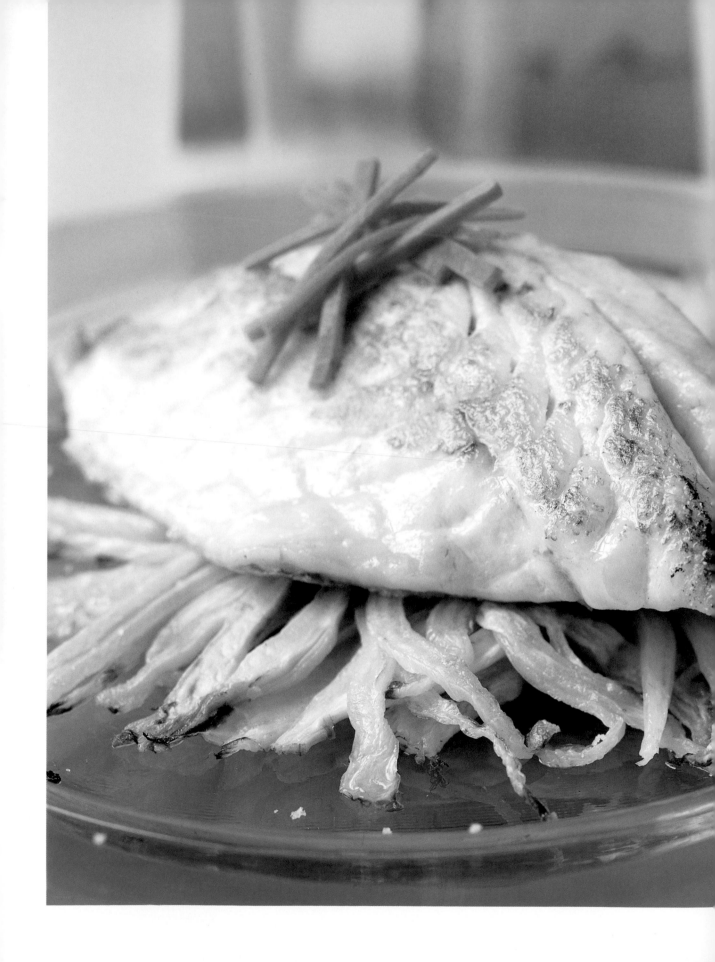

This chapter contains recipes that have been chosen to alleviate many of the symptoms experienced during the menopause. **You may be surprised to learn that simple changes to your diet can make a difference**. Many people are afraid that healthy eating will be time-consuming and will mean cutting out the foods that they enjoy. This certainly does not have to be the case, as **the recipes included in this chapter use fresh, readily available produce, they are simple to prepare and are delicious too**. There are plenty of recipes to choose from including soups, stir-fries, salads, pasta and risottos.

Each recipe has been nutritionally analysed to include the calories and kilojoules, grams of protein, carbohydrate, saturated fat and fibre.

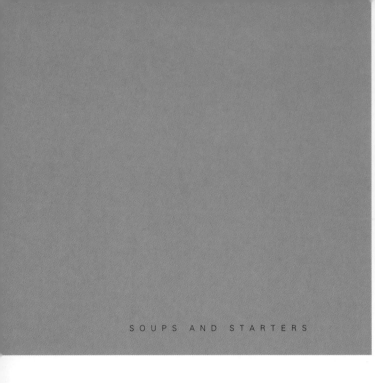
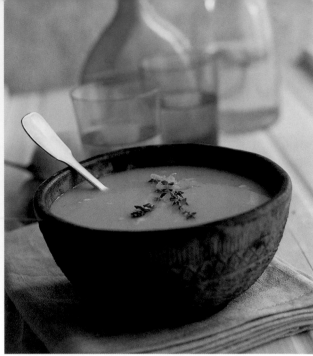

pumpkin and lemon soup

Serves 6 – Preparation time: 15 minutes – Cooking time: 40 minutes

Per serving – Energy 204 kcals/845 kJ · Protein 3 g · Carbohydrate 13 g · Fat 16 g · Saturated fat 10 g · Fibre 2 g

✔	alcohol free
✔	citrus free
	dairy free
✔	gluten free
✔	wheat free

25 g   **(1 oz) butter**
1   **large onion, sliced**
500 g   **(1 lb) pumpkin, peeled,**
    deseeded and cut into chunks
250 g   **(8 oz) potatoes, sliced**
1   **small garlic clove, crushed**
1   **thyme sprig, plus extra to garnish**
1.2   **litres (2 pints) chicken stock**
    juice of 1 lemon
150 ml   **(¼ pint) double cream**
    salt and pepper

1   Heat the butter in a large heavy saucepan, add the onion and cook over a gentle heat until soft and transparent. Add the pumpkin, potatoes, garlic and thyme. Cover the pan and cook slowly for 20 minutes, or until the vegetables are soft.

2   Pour in the stock, with salt and pepper to taste. Bring to the boil and simmer for 10 minutes. Remove and discard the thyme sprig.

3   Purée the soup in a food processor or blender or rub through a sieve. Squeeze in the lemon juice. Stir in the cream and reheat without boiling, then pour into warm bowls. Serve garnished with a thyme sprig. Alternatively, reserve a little of the cream and swirl it over the soup in the bowls.

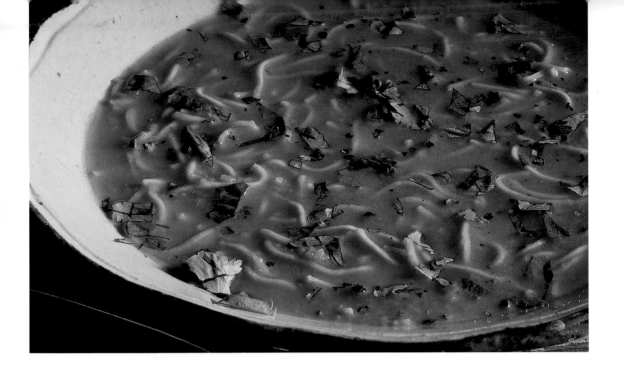

carrot and coriander noodle soup

Serves 4 – Preparation time: 10 minutes – Cooking time: about 40 minutes

Per serving – Energy 163 kcals/682 kJ · Protein 3 g · Carbohydrate 29 g · Fat 5 g · Saturated fat 1 g · Fibre 6 g

1	tablespoon vegetable oil
1	onion, chopped
750 g	(1½ lb) carrots, finely chopped
1	teaspoon ground coriander
150 ml	(¼ pint) orange juice
1 litre	(1¾ pints) hot vegetable stock
50 g	(2 oz) dried egg thread noodles
3	tablespoons chopped coriander
	salt and pepper

alcohol free	✔
citrus free	
dairy free	✔
gluten free	
wheat free	

1 Heat the oil in a large saucepan and fry the onion for 3 minutes until softened. Add the carrots, stir in the coriander and fry for 5 minutes, stirring occasionally. Add the orange juice and 900 ml (1½ pints) of the stock and bring to the boil. Lower the heat and simmer, partially covered, for 30 minutes.

2 Meanwhile, bring a large saucepan of water to the boil. Add the noodles, stir well and then cover the pan. Remove from the heat and set aside for 6 minutes. Drain the noodles, then snip them into 2.5 cm (1 inch) lengths. Set the noodles aside.

3 Purée the soup in batches in a food processor or blender. Return it to the rinsed saucepan and add the noodles. Stir in a little more stock if necessary. Add the chopped coriander, with salt and pepper to taste. Simmer the soup for 1 minute or until heated through, then serve.

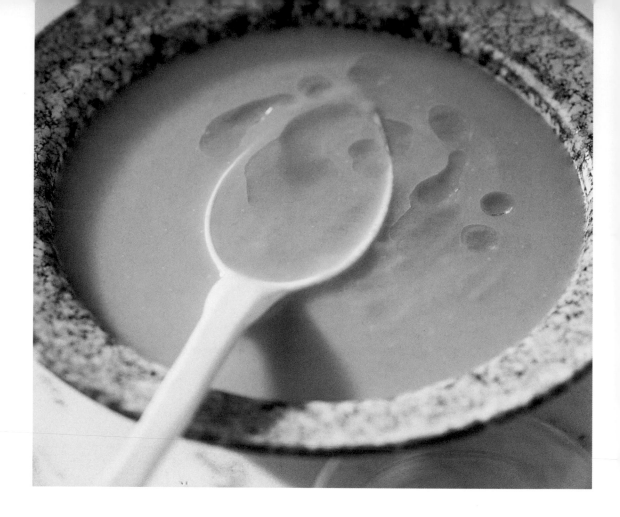

carrot and sage soup

Serves 6 – Preparation time: 15 minutes – Cooking time: about 1 hour

Per serving – Energy 87 kcals/363 kJ · Protein 1 g · Carbohydrate 12 g · Fat 4 g · Saturated fat 2 g · Fibre 4 g

✔	alcohol free
✔	citrus free
	dairy free
✔	gluten free
✔	wheat free

25 g (1 oz) butter
1 large onion, finely chopped
750 g (1½ lb) carrots, thinly sliced
900 ml (1½ pints) vegetable stock
1 tablespoon chopped sage leaves
salt and pepper
sage sprigs, to garnish (optional)

1 Melt the butter in a large heavy pan, add the onion and fry gently until soft but not golden, then add the carrots and stock. Season with salt and pepper. Bring to the boil and simmer, uncovered, for about 30 minutes.

2 Purée the soup in a food processor or blender until smooth, then return to the rinsed pan and add the chopped sage. Bring to the boil and simmer for another 15 minutes.

3 Serve the soup garnished with sage sprigs, if you like.

japanese miso soup with tofu

Serves 4 – Preparation time: 15 minutes – Cooking time: about 45 minutes

Per serving – Energy 52 kcals/216 kJ · Protein 6 g · Carbohydrate 2 g · Fat 2 g · Saturated fat 0 g · Fibre 1 g

2	**tablespoons red or white miso**
1	**small leek**
125 g	**(4 oz) firm tofu**
1	**tablespoon wakame seaweed**

Dashi Stock:

15 g	**(1½ oz) kombu seaweed**
1.8	**litres (3 pints) water**
2	**tablespoons dried tuna (bonito) flakes**

To Serve:
bunch of chives
pepper

alcohol free	✔
citrus free	✔
dairy free	✔
gluten free	✔
wheat free	✔

1 First make the dashi. Wipe the kombu seaweed with a damp cloth and put it into a saucepan with the water. Bring to a simmer, skimming away any scum that rises to the surface. When the soup is clear, add 1½ table-spoons of the dried tuna flakes and simmer, uncovered, for 20 minutes. Remove the pan from the heat and add the remaining dried tuna flakes. Set aside for 5 minutes, then strain the dashi and return to the pan.

2 Mix the miso with a little of the warm stock and add 1 tablespoon at a time to the remaining stock, stirring constantly until the miso has dissolved. Remove from the heat until ready to serve.

3 Cut the leek into fine julienne strips and the tofu into small squares. Warm the miso soup and add the leek and tofu with the wakame seaweed.

4 Blanch the chives, tie into a bundle and float on top of the soup and sprinkle with pepper. Serve immediately.

chilled fresh fruit soup

Serves 6 – Preparation time: 10 minutes, plus chilling

Per serving – Energy 293 kcals/1240 kJ · Protein 3 g · Carbohydrate 73 g · Fat 1 g · Saturated fat 0 g · Fibre 6 g

2	**dessert apples, peeled, quartered and cored**
6	**bananas, roughly chopped**
500 g	**(1 lb) strawberries**
375 g	**(12 oz) pears, peeled, quartered and cored**
1	**litre (1¾ pints) fresh orange juice**
2	**tablespoons fresh lemon juice**
300 ml	**(½ pint) fresh grapefruit juice**
5–6	**tablespoons clear honey**
	mint sprigs or strawberries, to garnish

alcohol free	✔
citrus free	
dairy free	✔
gluten free	✔
wheat free	✔

1 Place all the fruit in a food processor or blender with 300 ml (½ pint) of the orange juice and blend until very smooth. Add the lemon juice, grapefruit juice and honey. Blend again, in batches if necessary, until the mixture is smooth.

2 Pour the soup into a large bowl, stir in the remaining orange juice and cover the bowl loosely. Chill in the refrigerator for 3–4 hours.

3 Pour the chilled soup into 6 chilled bowls and garnish each one with a mint sprig or a strawberry.

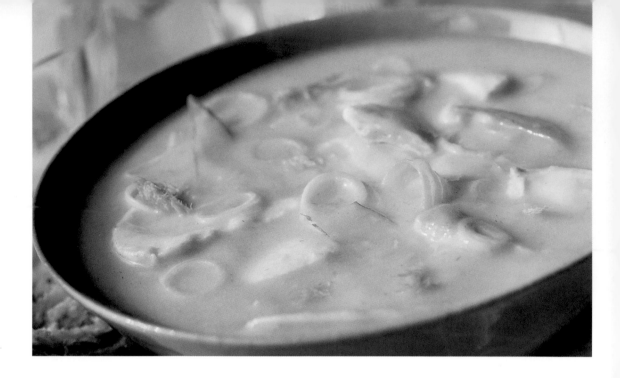

haddock and fennel soup

Serves 4 – Preparation time: 15 minutes – Cooking time: 25–30 minutes

Per serving – Energy 208 kcals/870 kJ · Protein 15 g · Carbohydrate 18 g · Fat 9 g · Saturated fat 5 g · Fibre 2 g

✔ alcohol free
✔ citrus free
dairy free
✔ gluten free
✔ wheat free

25 g	(1 oz) butter or margarine
250 g	(8 oz) fennel bulbs, thinly sliced, leaves reserved for garnish
1	leek, white part only, trimmed, cleaned and sliced
600 ml	(1 pint) fish stock
1	bay leaf
300 g	(10 oz) potatoes, thinly sliced
250 g	(8 oz) haddock fillets, skinned
300 ml	(½ pint) milk
½	teaspoon white pepper
	salt

1 Melt the butter or margarine in a saucepan. Add the fennel and leek slices and simmer for 5 minutes or until soft. Add the stock, bay leaf and potatoes. Bring to the boil, then lower the heat and simmer, covered, for 10–15 minutes or until the vegetables are tender. Remove and discard the bay leaf.

2 In another saucepan, combine the haddock with the milk and white pepper. Bring to the boil, then lower the heat and simmer, covered, for 5 minutes. Leave to stand with the lid on for a further 5 minutes, then break the fish into large flakes.

3 Put 300 ml (½ pint) of the fennel mixture in a food processor or blender and purée until smooth. Return the purée to the saucepan and add the milk and fish mixture. Stir well and heat thoroughly without boiling. Serve in warmed bowls, garnished with the reserved finely chopped fennel leaves.

lobster and corn chowder

Serves 4 – Preparation time: 40 minutes (if preparing the lobster yourself) **– Cooking time: about 1 hour**

Per serving – Energy 647 kcals/2727 kJ · Protein 43 g · Carbohydrate 67 g · Fat 24 g · Saturated fat 11 g · Fibre 8 g

2	lobsters, 750 g (1½ lb) each
25 g	(1 oz) butter
1	onion, finely chopped
1	carrot, finely chopped
1	celery stick, finely chopped
1	thyme sprig
1	parsley sprig
2	bay leaves
1	litre (1¾ pints) water
	Chowder:
200 g	(7 oz) canned sweetcorn kernels, drained
25 g	(1 oz) butter
1	small onion, chopped
1	small garlic clove, crushed
50 g	(2 oz) streaky bacon, cut into small strips
300 ml	(½ pint) semi-skimmed milk
150 ml	(¼ pint) single cream
1 kg	(2 lb) potatoes, cut into 1.5 cm (¾ inch) cubes
	pinch of cayenne pepper
4	tomatoes, skinned, deseeded and chopped
	salt and pepper

1 Cut the lobsters in half lengthways, remove and discard the green tomalley, gills and intestinal vein running along the back. Smash the claws, remove the meat and set aside. Cut the remaining meat into small pieces and set aside. Place the shells in a plastic bag and, using a rolling pin, smash into small pieces.

2 Melt the butter in a large saucepan over a low heat, add the onion, carrot and celery and cook, without colouring, for 8–10 minutes until softened. Add the herbs, water and the broken shells. Bring to the boil, then reduce the heat and simmer for 30 minutes. Strain through a fine sieve into a bowl.

3 To make the chowder, set aside one-third of the corn kernels. Place the remaining corn kernels in a food processor with the lobster broth and blend until smooth.

4 Melt the butter in a large flameproof casserole, add the onion and garlic and cook gently, without colouring, for 5 minutes. Add the bacon and cook until lightly golden.

5 Add the corn purée, milk, cream, potatoes and reserved corn. Bring to the boil, then reduce the heat and simmer for 10–15 minutes. Season to taste with salt, pepper and cayenne. Stir in the tomatoes and lobster meat and heat through gently.

alcohol free	✔
citrus free	✔
dairy free	
gluten free	✔
wheat free	✔

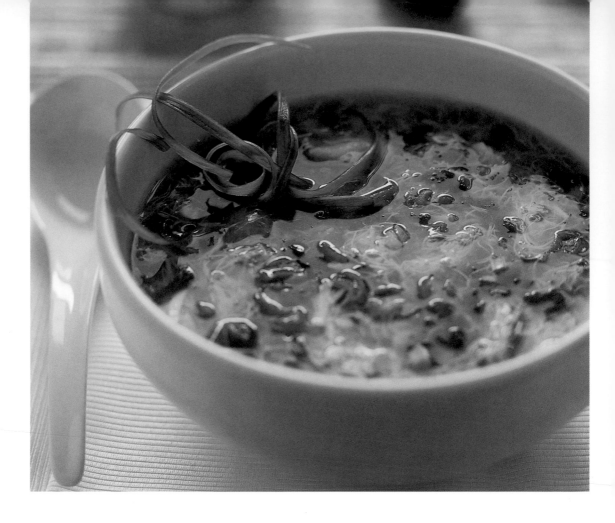

chinese crab soup

Serves 4 – Preparation time: 10 minutes – Cooking time: about 20 minutes

Per serving – Energy 90 kcals/380 kJ · Protein 8 g · Carbohydrate 9 g · Fat 2 g · Saturated fat 0 g · Fibre 1 g

	alcohol free
✔	citrus free
✔	dairy free
✔	gluten free
✔	wheat free

1 litre (1¾ pints) chicken stock
2.5 cm (1 inch) piece of root ginger,
very finely chopped
2 ripe tomatoes, skinned,
deseeded and very finely chopped
½ small red or green chilli,
deseeded and very finely chopped
2 tablespoons Chinese rice wine
or dry sherry
1 tablespoon rice wine vinegar
or white wine or cider vinegar
½ teaspoon sugar
1 tablespoon cornflour
about 150 g (5 oz) white crab meat,
defrosted and drained thoroughly
if frozen
salt and pepper
2 thinly sliced spring onions, to garnish

1 Put the stock into a large saucepan with the ginger, tomatoes, chilli, rice wine or sherry, vinegar and sugar. Bring to the boil, cover the pan and simmer for about 10 minutes.

2 Blend the cornflour to a paste with a little cold water, then pour it into the soup and stir to mix. Simmer, stirring, for 12 minutes until the soup thickens.

3 Add the crab meat, stir gently to mix, then heat through for 2–3 minutes. Taste the soup and add salt and pepper if necessary. Serve piping hot, sprinkled with the sliced spring onions.

raindrop soup

Serves 4 – Preparation time: 5 minutes – Cooking time: 10 minutes

Per serving – Energy 64 kcals/268 kJ · Protein 8 g · Carbohydrate 7 g · Fat 1 g · Saturated fat 0 g · Fibre 0 g

1	litre (1¾ pints) chicken stock
2	tablespoons Chinese rice wine or dry sherry
200 g	(7 oz) canned water chestnuts, drained and very thinly sliced into rounds
4	spring onions (white part only), very thinly sliced into rings
125 g	(4 oz) cooked peeled prawns
	salt and pepper
	a few drops of sesame oil, to finish

1 Pour the stock into a large saucepan and bring to the boil over a high heat. Stir in the rice wine or sherry, then add the water chestnuts and spring onions and simmer for 2 minutes.

2 Turn the heat down to low and add the prawns. Heat through gently for 1–2 minutes, then taste and add salt and pepper if necessary. Stir in a few drops of sesame oil before serving.

alcohol free	
citrus free	✔
dairy free	✔
gluten free	✔
wheat free	✔

mulligatawny soup

Serves 6 – Preparation time: 25 minutes – Cooking time: 30–40 minutes

Per serving – 317 kcals/1333 kJ · Protein 22 g · Carbohydrate 33 g · Fat 12 g · Saturated fat 3 g · Fibre 4 g

2	garlic cloves, finely chopped
2.5 cm	(1 inch) piece of root ginger
1	onion, roughly chopped
25 g	(1 oz) butter
2	tablespoons vegetable oil
1	tablespoon ground turmeric
2	teaspoons ground coriander
1	tablespoon Madras curry paste or powder
175 g	(6 oz) red lentils
75 g	(3 oz) long-grain rice
1.8	litres (3 pints) chicken stock
1	green dessert apple, chopped
2	chicken breasts, cooked and shredded

To Garnish:

	oil, for frying
2	onions, thinly sliced
6	tablespoons natural yogurt
1	large green chilli, sliced

1 Place the garlic, ginger and onion in a food processor or blender and process for 12 minutes, or until finely chopped.

2 Heat the butter and oil in a large heavy pan over a moderate heat. Add the processed garlic mixture, turmeric, coriander and curry paste or powder. Cook for 45 minutes, stirring occasionally, until the onion is brown. Add the lentils and rice and stir to combine. Cook for 2–3 minutes.

3 Add the stock and chopped apple to the pan and stir gently to combine. Bring slowly to the boil and boil for 3 minutes, then reduce the heat and simmer for 20 minutes, or until the lentils and rice are tender. Stir in the chicken, cover and cook for 3 minutes.

4 To make the garnish, heat the oil. Separate the onions into rings and shallow-fry in small batches over a moderate heat until brown and crisp. Drain on kitchen paper.

5 Serve the soup in individual bowls, topped with a spoonful of yogurt and garnished with onion rings and a few chilli slices.

alcohol free	✔
citrus free	✔
dairy free	
gluten free	✔
wheat free	✔

tempura

Serves 4 – Preparation time: 30 minutes – Cooking time: 20–30 minutes

Per serving – Energy 483 kcals/2029 kJ · Protein 35 g · Carbohydrate 48 g · Fat 16 g · Saturated fat 2 g · Fibre 5 g

900 ml (1½ pints) oil, for deep-frying

12 raw tiger prawns,
   peeled, but with tails left on

500 g (1 lb) plaice or sole fillets,
   skinned and cut into small pieces

8 button mushrooms

1 bunch of spring onions,
   cut into 3.5 cm (1½ inch) lengths

1 red pepper, cored, deseeded and sliced

1 green pepper, cored, deseeded
   and sliced

1 large onion, cut into wedges

½ small cauliflower, broken into florets

½ small aubergine, thinly sliced
   chives, to garnish

Batter:

1 egg

150 ml (¼ pint) water

125 g (4 oz) plain flour

50 g (2 oz) cornflour
   pinch of salt

Dipping Sauce:

300 ml (½ pint) canned chicken consommé

4 tablespoons sweet vermouth or sherry

4 tablespoons light soy sauce

1 To make the batter, lightly beat the egg in a large bowl. Beat in the water until frothy. Sift together the flour, cornflour and salt and fold in gradually.

2 Heat the oil in a wok. Dip the prawns, fish pieces and vegetables into the batter, then deep-fry in batches, until golden. Drain on kitchen paper; keep warm.

3 To make the dipping sauce, gently heat all the ingredients in a saucepan, then transfer to a warmed bowl. Serve immediately.

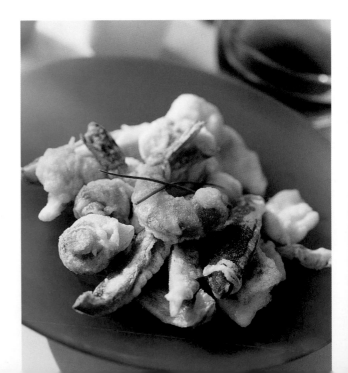

chilled stuffed artichokes

Serves 4 – Preparation time: 30 minutes – Cooking time: about 35 minutes

Per serving – Energy 193 kcals/809 kJ · Protein 12 g · Carbohydrate 28 g · Fat 4 g · Saturated fat 1 g · Fibre 1 g

4	artichokes, stems trimmed and top third of leaves removed
1	tablespoon fresh lemon juice
½	quantity Steamed Vegetables with Ginger (see page 110), chilled

Sauce:

150 g	(5 oz) tofu, drained
4	tablespoons tomato purée
4	tablespoons horseradish sauce
2	teaspoons fresh lemon juice
2	teaspoons white vinegar
¼	teaspoon grated lemon rind
½	teaspoon onion salt
½	teaspoon sugar
	few drops of Tabasco sauce
	freshly ground white pepper, to taste

1 Place the artichokes and lemon juice in a deep saucepan and add boiling water to cover. Cover and cook for 30 minutes, or until one of the outer artichoke leaves pulls off easily. Remove from the pan, turn upside down to drain, then refrigerate to cool.

2 Remove the central choke of each artichoke and fill with some chilled steamed vegetables.

3 To make the sauce, place all the ingredients in a food processor or blender and purée. Pour some sauce over each artichoke to serve.

alcohol free	✔
citrus free	
dairy free	✔
gluten free	✔
wheat free	✔

baked stuffed mushrooms

Serves 4 – Preparation time: 10 minutes – Cooking time: 25 minutes

Per serving – Energy 166 kcals/692 kJ · Protein 6 g · Carbohydrate 11 g · Fat 11 g · Saturated fat 3 g · Fibre 2 g

4	large field mushrooms
1	small onion, very finely chopped
50 g	(2 oz) mini macaroni, cooked
25 g	(1 oz) walnuts, chopped
1	tablespoon chopped parsley
25 g	(1 oz) Cheddar cheese, cubed
1	tablespoon tomato purée
1	egg, beaten
1	tablespoon olive oil
	salt and pepper

1 Chop the mushroom stalks finely and set aside. Peel the mushrooms, if blemished, and grill for 5 minutes until just softened. Remove and set aside.

2 Put the chopped onion into a large bowl. Add the chopped mushroom stalks, cooked macaroni, walnuts, parsley, cheese and tomato purée. Mix well, then add enough of the beaten egg to bind the mixture. Add salt and pepper to taste.

3 Divide the filling between the mushrooms, mounding the mixture up with a spoon. Drizzle over a little olive oil. Arrange the filled mushrooms, well apart on a grill pan.

4 Grill for 15–20 minutes until the top of the stuffing is crisp and has started to char at the edges.

alcohol free	✔
citrus free	✔
dairy free	
gluten free	
wheat free	

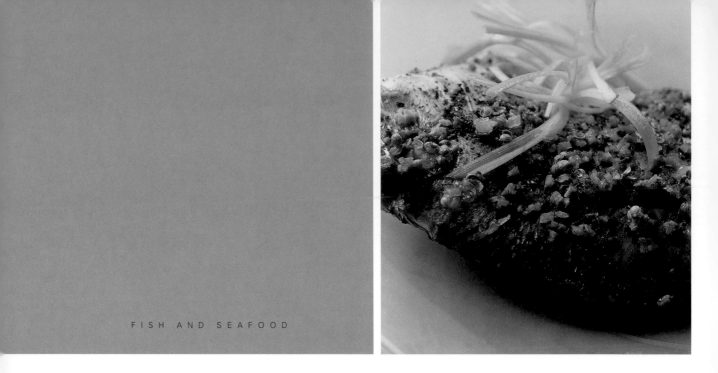

steamed spiced fish

Serves 6 – Preparation time: 10 minutes, plus standing – Cooking time: 15–20 minutes
Per serving – Energy 210 kcals/880 kJ · Protein 33 g · Carbohydrate 1 g · Fat 8 g · Saturated fat 1 g · Fibre 0 g

✔	alcohol free
	citrus free
✔	dairy free
✔	gluten free
✔	wheat free

1.5 kg	**(3 lb) whole bass, bream or grey mullet, cleaned**
1	**tablespoon sea salt**
1	**tablespoon cumin seeds, lightly crushed**
5 cm	**(2 inch) piece of root ginger, finely chopped**
2	**tablespoons fresh lemon juice**
2	**tablespoons olive oil**
2–3	**garlic cloves, finely chopped**
1	**tablespoon coriander seeds, crushed spring onion curls, to garnish pepper**

1 Rinse the fish in cold water, then rub it all over with salt and lots of black pepper. Leave to stand, covered, at room temperature for 30 minutes.

2 Put a grill rack into a roasting pan and pour in 2.5 cm (1 inch) boiling water. Set over a low heat so the liquid is gently simmering.

3 Transfer the fish to a heatproof serving plate, discarding any liquid which may have collected around it. Sprinkle on the cumin seeds and ginger, then put the plate on to the rack. Cover the whole roasting pan with foil, pressing it around the edges to form as close a seal as possible, then cook for 15–20 minutes until the fish flakes easily. Test it with the point of a sharp knife near the gills. Take off the heat, remove the foil, and sprinkle over the lemon juice.

4 Heat the oil in a small frying pan. Stir-fry the garlic and coriander seeds over a high heat for about 1 minute. Pour the sizzling oil over the fish, garnish with spring onion curls and serve.

japanese tofu and fish hotpot

Serves 6 – Preparation time: 30 minutes, plus soaking – Cooking time: about 30 minutes

Per serving – Energy 406 kcals/1699 kJ · Protein 35 g · Carbohydrate 44 g · Fat 9 g · Saturated fat 2 g · Fibre 1 g

6	**Chinese cabbage leaves**
125 g	**(4 oz) sugar snap peas**
300 g	**(10 oz) cellophane noodles (saifan)**
2	**boneless, skinless chicken thighs**
125 g	**(4 oz) sea bream fillets**
125 g	**(4 oz) mackerel fillets**
1.8	**litres (3 pints) fish stock**
5	**tablespoons mirin**
	(sweet Japanese rice wine)
2.5 cm	**(1 inch) piece of root ginger, grated**
6	**spring onions, chopped**
1	**tablespoon soy sauce**
175 g	**(6 oz) clams**
125 g	**(4 oz) small cooked, peeled prawns**
250 g	**(8 oz) firm tofu, cubed**
75 g	**(3 oz) watercress, chopped**
125 g	**(4 oz) enoki or shiitake**
	mushrooms, halved

Red Maple Relish:

75 g	**(3 oz) daikon radish**
2	**small chillies**

alcohol free	✔
citrus free	✔
dairy free	✔
gluten free	
wheat free	

1 Blanch the cabbage and sugar snap peas in boiling water for 1 minute, then drain and refresh in cold water. Shred the cabbage.

2 Place the noodles in a large bowl, cover with hot water and leave to soak for about 10 minutes or until softened.

3 Slice the chicken into cubes and the fish into 5 cm (2 inch) pieces. Put the stock, mirin, ginger, spring onions and soy sauce into a large pan and bring to the boil. Reduce the heat to a simmer, add the chicken and simmer for 8–10 minutes.

4 To make the red maple relish, make two deep holes in the large end of the daikon with a chopstick and insert the chillies. Grate the daikon and chillies together very finely. Then put them in a mortar and pound with a pestle.

5 Add the clams, prawns, sliced fish, soaked noodles and tofu to the simmering hotpot and take it to the table. Simmer for a further 6–8 minutes or until the clams open and the fish has cooked. Discard any clams that remain closed.

6 Arrange the cabbage, blanched sugar snap peas, watercress, mushrooms and red maple relish on a serving platter and serve with the hotpot. Add the watercress and mushrooms to the hotpot and cook for 1 minute. Place a few items in each serving bowl and ladle some stock over the top. Allow diners to help themselves to more as they eat

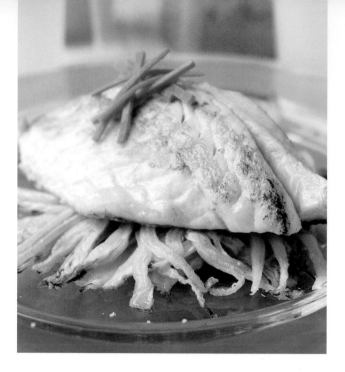

sea bass with fennel

Serves 4 – Preparation time: 5 minutes – Cooking time: 45–50 minutes

Per serving – Energy 384 kcals/1600 kJ · Protein 44 g · Carbohydrate 2 g · Fat 22 g · Saturated fat 3 g · Fibre 2 g

✔	alcohol free
✔	citrus free
✔	dairy free
✔	gluten free
✔	wheat free

2 **large fennel bulbs**
6 **tablespoons olive oil**
8 **tablespoons water**
2 **sea bass, about 500 g (1 lb) each, filleted**
salt and pepper
carrot matchsticks, to garnish

1 Cut the fennel bulbs lengthways into 1 cm (½ inch) slices. Pour the oil into a wok, add the fennel and water and bring to the boil. Cover and simmer for 30 minutes, until the fennel is very tender, stirring occasionally.

2 Remove the lid, season the fennel with salt and pepper and boil until all the water has evaporated and the fennel is golden brown. Transfer to a warmed plate and keep hot.

3 Season the fish with salt and pepper, add to the wok and baste with the hot oil. Cover and cook for 7–8 minutes. Turn the fish over, baste again and cook for about 5 more minutes.

4 Arrange the fennel on a warmed serving dish, place the fish on the fennel and pour the cooking juices around and over the fish. Serve immediately, garnished with carrot matchsticks.

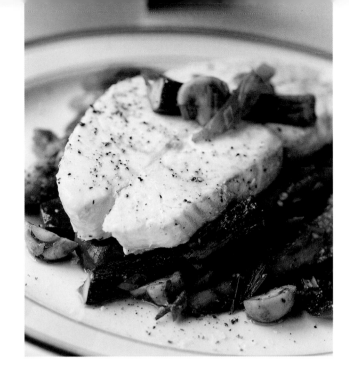

halibut on a bed of vegetables

Serves 2 – Preparation time: 20 minute – Cooking time: about 25 minutes

Per serving – Energy 382 kcals/1594 kJ · Protein 30 g · Carbohydrate 9 g · Fat 26 g · Saturated fat 4 g · Fibre 4 g

2	tablespoons olive oil
½	red pepper, cored, deseeded and roughly chopped
½	green pepper, cored, deseeded and roughly chopped
50 g	(2 oz) mushrooms, sliced
1	courgette, sliced lengthways into 3 cm (1½ inch) pieces
½	aubergine, sliced lengthways into 3 cm (1½ inch) pieces
2	tomatoes, skinned and chopped
1	tablespoon tomato purée
2	halibut steaks, about 150–175 g (5–6 oz) each
25 g	(1 oz) butter
2	tablespoons chopped mixed parsley, tarragon and chives
	salt and pepper

1 Heat the oil in a large saucepan, add the red and green peppers, mushrooms, courgette, aubergine, tomatoes and tomato purée and fry for 15–20 minutes over a moderate heat, stirring occasionally.

2 Meanwhile, line a baking sheet with a large piece of foil, allowing sufficient to fold over comfortably. Place the fish on the foil, dot with butter, sprinkle with 1 tablespoon of the herbs and season with salt and pepper. Fold the foil loosely over the fish and bake in a preheated oven, 200°C (400°F), Gas Mark 6, for 18–20 minutes until cooked through.

3 When the fish and vegetables are cooked, season to taste and add more herbs or tomato purée if necessary. Spoon the vegetables on to warmed plates and put the halibut on top. Serve immediately, sprinkled with the remaining herbs.

alcohol free	✔
citrus free	✔
dairy free	
gluten free	✔
wheat free	✔

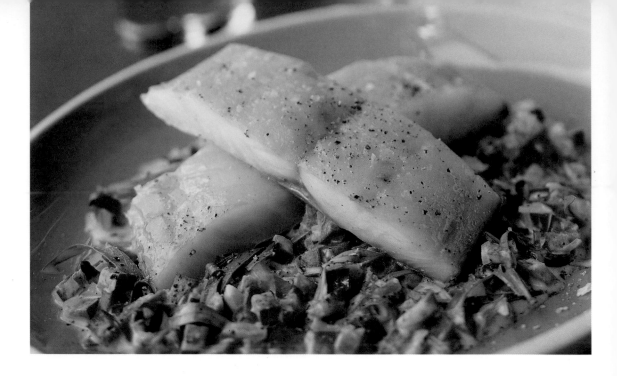

smoked haddock with red pepper sauce

Serves 2 – Preparation time: 10 minutes – Cooking time: about 25 minutes

Per serving – Energy 373 kcals/1568 kJ · Protein 42 g · Carbohydrate 19 g · Fat 15 g · Saturated fat 2 g · Fibre 2 g

✔	alcohol free
✔	citrus free
	dairy free
✔	gluten free
✔	wheat free

2	**smoked haddock fillets**
300 ml	**(½ pint) semi-skimmed milk**
1	**tablespoon olive oil**
2	**shallots, finely chopped**
1	**garlic clove, crushed**
2	**large red peppers, cored, deseeded, and finely chopped**
200 ml	**(7 fl oz) half-fat crème fraîche**
1	**tablespoon chopped tarragon, plus extra to garnish**
	salt and pepper

1 Put the haddock fillets into a shallow pan, add the milk and poach for 5 minutes, or until done. Remove the haddock, cover and keep warm. Strain and reserve the milk.

2 Meanwhile, heat the oil in a frying pan, add the shallots and garlic and fry gently for 5 minutes until soft. Add the red peppers and cook gently for 7–8 minutes, stirring occasionally.

3 Put the crème fraîche into a bowl and stir in 4 table-spoons of the strained milk. Stir in the red pepper mixture (or purée it in a food processor if you would like a very smooth sauce). Return the mixture to the pan and add the tarragon. Season the sauce to taste with salt and pepper, then simmer for 10 minutes.

4 To serve, pour the sauce on to the plate and place the haddock on top. Sprinkle with pepper, garnish with tarragon and serve immediately.

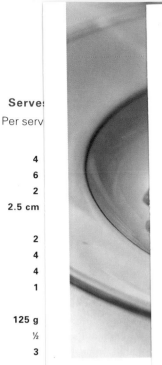

Serves
Per serv

4
6
2
2.5 cm

2
4
4
1

125 g
½
3

2
150 ml

cod baked with potatoes, onions and tomatoes

Serves 4 – Preparation time: 15 minutes – Cooking time: about 30 minutes

Per serving – Energy 430 kcals/1813 kJ · Protein 36 g · Carbohydrate 33 g · Fat 16 g · Saturated fat 4 g · Fibre 4 g

12	small new potatoes
1	tablespoon olive oil
4	cod fillets
2	tablespoons extra virgin olive oil
2	onions, finely chopped
1	garlic clove, crushed
1	tablespoon chopped oregano
425 g	(14 oz) can chopped tomatoes
125 ml	(4 fl oz) dry white wine or fish stock
75 g	(3 oz) fine breadcrumbs
50 g	(2 oz) grated Parmesan or Cheddar cheese
	salt and pepper
	chopped parsley, to garnish

1 Boil the potatoes until almost done. Cut them into thick slices and coat in olive oil. Arrange them around a greased ovenproof dish and place the fish in the centre.

2 Meanwhile, heat the extra virgin olive oil in a pan, add the onions and sauté for about 5 minutes until soft. Add the garlic and oregano and cook for 2–3 minutes. Add the tomatoes, wine or stock and salt and pepper to taste and simmer for a few minutes.

3 Spoon half of the tomato mixture over the potatoes and fish. Mix the remaining mixture with the breadcrumbs and cheese and then pour over the fish. Bake in a pre-heated oven, 200°C (400°F), Gas Mark 6, for 15 minutes or until the fish is cooked. Garnish with parsley.

alcohol free	
citrus free	✔
dairy free	
gluten free	
wheat free	

Per serving – En

4   tablespo
1 cm (½ inch)
      and fi
2   garlic cl
8   spring o
      sliced
1   carrot, p
8   celery st
375 g (12 oz) c
      into ti
2   red pepp
      and s
1   green pe
      and sl
1 kg (2 lb) lar
      celery le

      Glaze:
2   teaspoo
6   tablespo
2   tablespo
2   teaspoo
2   teaspoo
      salt and

sauté of scallops with mangetout

Serves 2 – Preparation time: 15 minutes – Cooking time: about 10 minutes

Per serving – Energy 344 kcals/1438 kJ · Protein 24 g · Carbohydrate 11 g · Fat 23 g · Saturated fat 3 g · Fibre 4 g

8	shelled scallops with coral
3	tablespoons vegetable oil
6	spring onions, thinly sliced diagonally
2.5 cm	(1 inch) piece of root ginger, finely chopped
175 g	(6 oz) mangetout, trimmed
1	garlic clove, crushed
1	tablespoon sesame oil
2	tablespoons soy sauce
½	teaspoon caster sugar
	pepper
	spring onions, to garnish

1 Slice the scallops thickly, detaching the corals and keeping them whole. Set the corals aside.

2 Heat 2 tablespoons of the vegetable oil in a wok over a moderate heat. Add the spring onions and ginger and stir-fry for a few seconds. Add the mangetout and garlic and stir-fry for 2 minutes, then tip the vegetable mixture into a bowl and set aside.

3 Heat the remaining vegetable oil with the sesame seed oil over a moderate heat. Add the sliced scallops and stir-fry for 3 minutes. Return the spring onion, ginger and mangetout mixture to the wok, add the reserved corals, soy sauce and sugar and increase the heat to high. Toss for 1–2 minutes or until all the ingredients are combined and piping hot. Season with pepper to taste and serve immediately, garnished with spring onions.

alcohol free	✔
citrus free	✔
dairy free	✔
gluten free	
wheat free	

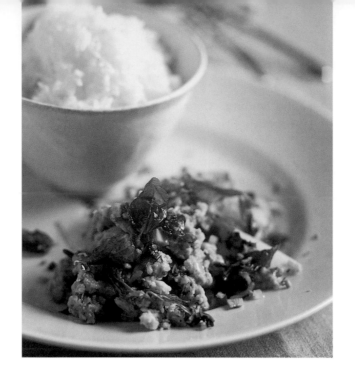

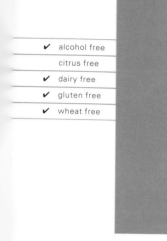

✔ alcohol free
citrus free
✔ dairy free
✔ gluten free
✔ wheat free

thai minced chicken with basil

✔ alcohol free
✔ citrus free
✔ dairy free
gluten free
wheat free

✔ alcol
✔ citru
✔ dairy
glute
whea

alcohol free
citrus free
✔ dairy free
gluten free
wheat free

Serves 2 – Preparation time: 6 minutes – Cooking time: 6 minutes

Per serving – Energy 399 kcals/1653 kJ · Protein 19 g · Carbohydrate 14 g · Fat 30 g · Saturated fat 5 g · Fibre 1 g

5	**small green chillies**
2	**garlic cloves**
2	**tablespoons oil**
125 g	**(4 oz) minced chicken**
1	**shallot, chopped**
25 g	**(1 oz) bamboo shoots**
25 g	**(1 oz) red pepper, cored, deseeded and chopped**
15 g	**(½ oz) carrot, diced**
1	**teaspoon palm sugar or light muscovado sugar**
3	**tablespoons Thai fish sauce or light soy sauce**
3	**tablespoons chicken stock**
15 g	**(½ oz) basil leaves, finely chopped rice, to serve**

Crispy Garlic, Shallot and Basil Garnish:

	groundnut oil, for deep-frying
25 g	**(1 oz) garlic, finely chopped**
25 g	**(1 oz) shallots, finely chopped**
25 g	**(1 oz) basil leaves**
1	**small red chilli, thinly sliced**

1 To make the garnish, heat the oil in a wok. When it is hot, add the garlic and stir for about 40 seconds. Remove with a slotted spoon, draining as much oil as possible back into the wok, then dry on kitchen paper. Repeat the process with the shallots, allowing 1½–2 minutes frying time. Then add the basil leaves and chilli to the oil and fry for about 1 minute. Remove with a slotted spoon and drain as before.

2 To cook the chicken, put the chillies and garlic into a mortar and pound with a pestle until well broken down.

3 Heat the oil in a wok, add the pounded chillies and garlic and stir-fry for 30 seconds. Add the remaining ingredients and cook, stirring, for 4 minutes over a moderate heat. Increase the heat to high and stir vigorously for 30 seconds.

4 Transfer to a warmed dish and serve with rice and sprinkled with the crispy garlic, shallot and basil garnish.

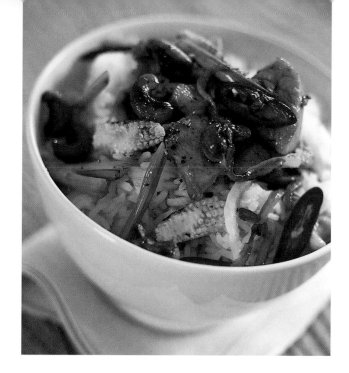

stir-fried chicken with cashew nuts and baby corn

Serves 2 – Preparation time: 10 minutes – Cooking time: about 7 minutes

Per serving – Energy 414 kcals/1726 kJ · Protein 23 g · Carbohydrate 22 g · Fat 26 g · Saturated fat 4 g · Fibre 0 g

2	**tablespoons oil**
125 g	**(4 oz) chicken, skinned and cut into bite-sized pieces**
¼	**onion, sliced**
50 g	**(2 oz) baby corn, diagonally sliced**
50 g	**(2 oz) cashew nuts**
125 ml	**(4 fl oz) light soy sauce**
4	**tablespoons chicken stock**
4	**teaspoons palm sugar or light muscovado sugar**
15 g	**(½ oz) spring onion, diagonally sliced**
	pepper
1	**large red chilli, diagonally sliced, to garnish**

1 Heat the oil in a wok, add the chicken, onion, baby corn and cashew nuts. Stir-fry over a high heat for 3 minutes.

2 Reduce the heat and stir in the soy sauce, then add the stock, sugar and spring onion and season with pepper. Raise the heat and stir-fry for another 2 minutes.

3 Turn on to a serving dish or into 2 individual bowls, sprinkle with sliced chilli and serve.

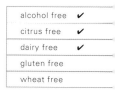

alcohol free	✔
citrus free	✔
dairy free	✔
gluten free	
wheat free	

chicken with sizzling garlic sauce

Serves 2 – Preparation time: 10–15 minutes, plus marinating – Cooking time: 10 minutes

Per serving – Energy 526 kcals/2207 kJ · Protein 31 g · Carbohydrate 50 g · Fat 24 g · Saturated fat 5 g · Fibre 1 g

	alcohol free
✔	citrus free
✔	dairy free
✔	gluten free
✔	wheat free

2 boneless, skinless chicken breasts, total weight 250–300 g (8–10 oz), cut into thin strips
1 small egg
2 garlic cloves, crushed
  about 4 tablespoons cornflour
  about 175 ml (6 fl oz) groundnut oil, for frying
  salt and pepper
  a few drops of chilli oil (optional), to serve

Garlic Sauce:
4 spring onions (white part only), finely shredded
2 garlic cloves, finely chopped
200 ml (7 fl oz) hot chicken stock
4 tablespoons Chinese rice wine or dry sherry
1 teaspoon cornflour

To Garnish:
½ tablespoon finely chopped red pepper
½ tablespoon finely chopped green pepper
1 tablespoon chopped coriander (optional)

1 Put the chicken breasts between clingfilm and pound them with the bottom of a saucepan to flatten them. Remove the clingfilm and cut the chicken into strips about 2.5 cm (1 inch) wide.

2 Beat the egg in a bowl with the crushed garlic and plenty of salt and pepper. Dip the chicken strips in the egg mixture, then place them in a single layer on a plate and dredge them with cornflour. Put the plate in the refrigerator for about 1 hour, or longer if you have the time.

3 Heat the oil in a wok until very hot, but not smoking. Immerse the chicken pieces in the hot oil in a single layer. Fry for about 3 minutes or until the chicken is golden, turning once. Remove with a slotted spoon and keep hot in a warmed bowl. Repeat with the remaining chicken.

4 Very carefully pour off all but about 1 teaspoon of the hot oil from the wok. Return the wok to a low heat and make the sauce. Put the spring onions, chopped garlic, stock and rice wine or sherry in the wok. Increase the heat to high and bring to the boil, stirring.

5 Blend the cornflour to a paste with a little cold water, then pour it into the wok and stir to mix. Simmer, stirring, for 1–2 minutes until the sauce thickens, then pour it over the chicken. Garnish with the red and green pepper and chopped coriander, if using, and sprinkle with a few drops of chilli oil, if liked. Serve immediately.

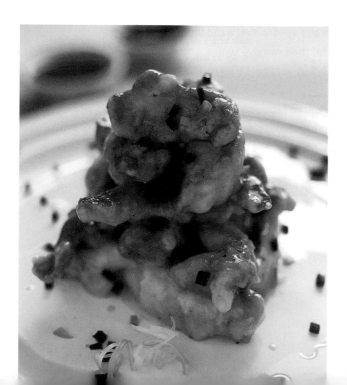

chicken and prawn kebabs

Serves 6 – Preparation time: 15 minutes, plus marinating – Cooking time: about 20 minutes

Per serving – Energy 250 kcals/1053 kJ · Protein 34 g · Carbohydrate 2 g · Fat 12 g · Saturated fat 2 g · Fibre 1 g

750 g	(1½ lb) boneless, skinless chicken breasts, cut into 2.5 cm (1 inch) cubes
20	cooked large prawns
1	small yellow or red pepper, cored, deseeded and cut into 2.5 cm (1 inch) squares
1	small green pepper, cored, deseeded and cut into 2.5 cm (1 inch) squares
	lime wedges, to garnish

Herb Marinade:

4	tablespoons sunflower oil
2	tablespoons lemon juice
1	teaspoon chopped marjoram
1	teaspoon chopped thyme
2	tablespoons chopped parsley
1	garlic clove, crushed
1	onion, finely chopped
	salt and pepper

1 Thread the chicken, prawns and peppers alternately on to presoaked bamboo or oiled metal skewers. Mix together all the ingredients for the herb marinade in a bowl with salt and pepper to taste. Place the skewers in a shallow dish and pour over the marinade. Turn the skewers to coat with the marinade. Cover and leave for 2 hours in a cool place, turning occasionally.

2 Remove the kebabs from the marinade, reserving the marinade. Cook the kebabs under a preheated moderate hot grill for about 20 minutes, turning and basting frequently with the reserved marinade.

3 Serve garnished with lime wedges.

alcohol free	✔
citrus free	
dairy free	✔
gluten free	✔
wheat free	✔

stir-fried chicken with pineapple

Serves 4 – Preparation time: 10 minutes – Cooking time: 12–14 minutes

Per serving – Energy 270 kcals/1136 kJ · Protein 11 g · Carbohydrate 22 g · Fat 16 g · Saturated fat 3 g · Fibre 2 g

	oil, for deep-frying
50 g	(2 oz) Japanese tempura flour or self-raising flour
75 ml	(3 fl oz) water
125 g	(4 oz) chicken, skinned and cut into bite-sized pieces
1	tablespoon groundnut oil
150 g	(5 oz) fresh pineapple, cut into chunks
1	tomato, cut into 8 pieces
1	tablespoon tomato purée
1	tablespoon palm sugar or light muscovado sugar
50 g	(2 oz) cashew nuts
1½	tablespoons light soy sauce

To Garnish:

alfalfa or bean sprouts

coriander sprigs

½	lime

1 Heat the oil for deep-frying in a wok and, while it is heating, mix the flour and water to make a coating batter.

2 When the oil is hot enough, coat half the chicken pieces in the batter and deep-fry them until they are golden brown. Remove them from the oil and drain on kitchen paper. Repeat with the remaining chicken.

3 Pour off the oil, wipe the wok with kitchen paper, then heat the groundnut oil. Add the pineapple, tomato, tomato purée, sugar and cashews and stir-fry for 2 minutes. Add the soy sauce and stir.

4 Serve the batter-coated chicken on the tomato and pineapple mixture, garnished with alfalfa or bean sprouts, coriander sprigs and ½ lime.

alcohol free	✔
citrus free	✔
dairy free	✔
gluten free	
wheat free	

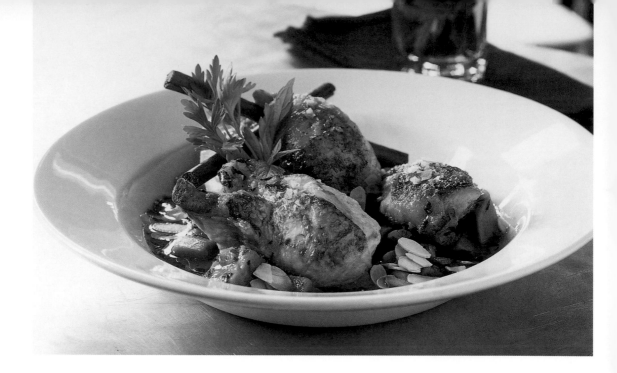

chicken, squash and sweet potato tagine

Serves 4 – Preparation time: 20 minutes – Cooking time: 1 hour

Per serving – Energy 465 kcals/1953 kJ · Protein 40 g · Carbohydrate 48 g · Fat 14 g · Saturated fat 3 g · Fibre 8 g

✔	alcohol free
✔	citrus free
✔	dairy free
✔	gluten free
✔	wheat free

2   **tablespoons olive oil**

700 g   **(1½ lb) boneless, skinless chicken**

2   **large onions, finely chopped**

4   **garlic cloves, crushed**

2   **cinnamon sticks, broken in half**

500 g   **(1 lb) sweet potatoes,**
    cut into small cubes

500 g   **(1 lb) squash or pumpkin,**
    cut into small cubes

    small handful of chopped mixed
    parsley and mint

300 ml   **(½ pint) chicken stock**

    salt and pepper

To Garnish:
flaked almonds
parsley sprigs
mint sprigs

1 Heat the oil in a large heavy casserole. Add the chicken in batches and brown evenly. Remove and keep warm. Add the onions to the casserole and cook until soft and lightly browned, adding the garlic and cinnamon when the onions are nearly done.

2 Stir in the sweet potatoes and squash or pumpkin, then return the chicken to the pan, add half of the parsley and mint and pour in the stock. Cover tightly and simmer very gently for about 45 minutes until the chicken and vegetables are tender.

3 Season to taste with salt and pepper, then add the remaining parsley and mint. Scatter over the almonds and serve garnished with parsley and mint sprigs.

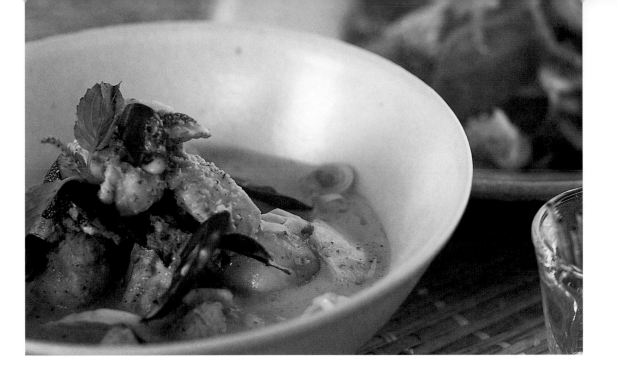

thai green chicken curry

Serves 2 – Preparation time: 5–7 minutes – Cooking time: 13–15 minutes

Per serving – Energy 230 kcals/969 kJ · Protein 18 g · Carbohydrate 17 g · Fat 11 g · Saturated fat 1 g · Fibre 2 g

1	tablespoon oil
1½	tablespoons ready-made green curry paste
4	tablespoons coconut milk
125 g	(4 oz) chicken breast, cut into bite-sized pieces
2	lime leaves, torn, or 2 strips lime rind
½	lemon grass stalk, cut in fine, oblique slices (optional)
50 g	(2 oz) bamboo shoots
3	small green aubergines, or 1 purple aubergine, chopped
50 g	(2 oz) courgettes, cut into diagonal chunks
1	large red chilli, diagonally sliced
6	tablespoons chicken stock
1	tablespoon palm sugar or light muscovado sugar
3	tablespoons Thai fish sauce or light soy sauce
	basil sprigs, to garnish

1 Heat the oil in a wok and stir in the curry paste. Cook for 30 seconds, then add the coconut milk and cook, stirring, for 1 minute.

2 Add the chicken, bring to a simmer, then add all the remaining ingredients. Simmer gently for 10 minutes, stirring occasionally.

3 Transfer the curry to a warmed serving bowl, garnish with basil sprigs and serve.

alcohol free	✔
citrus free	
dairy free	✔
gluten free	
wheat free	

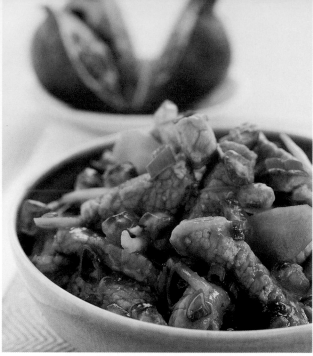

sweet and spicy pork with pomegranate

Serves 2 – Preparation time: 30 minutes – Cooking time: about 15 minutes

Per serving – Energy 553 kcals/2315 kJ · Protein 44 g · Carbohydrate 40 g · Fat 25 g · Saturated fat 7 g · Fibre 7 g

alcohol free	
citrus free	✔
dairy free	✔
gluten free	
wheat free	

1 pork fillet (tenderloin),
     weighing about 375 g (12 oz)
2 tablespoons groundnut oil
4–7 spring onions, roughly chopped
2.5 cm (1 inch) piece of root ginger,
     finely chopped
2 garlic cloves, finely chopped
2–3 carrots, very thinly
     sliced diagonally
125 g (4 oz) bean sprouts
     seeds of 1 pomegranate
     salt and pepper

Sauce:
4 tablespoons Chinese rice wine
     or dry sherry
2 tablespoons soy sauce,
     or more to taste
2 tablespoons chilli sauce,
     or more to taste
2 tablespoons clear honey
1 tablespoon tomato purée
2 teaspoons cornflour

1 Cut the pork fillet crossways into 2 cm (¾ inch) slices, then cut these slices crossways into 2–3 strips. Mix the sauce ingredients in a measuring jug, add cold water up to the 250 ml (8 fl oz) mark and stir well to mix.

2 Heat an empty wok until hot. Add the oil and heat until very hot. Add the spring onions, ginger and garlic and stir-fry over a moderate heat for 1 minute. Add the carrots and stir-fry for 1–2 minutes.

3 Increase the heat to high, add the pork and stir-fry for 5 minutes. Pour in the sauce mixture and bring to the boil, stirring constantly, then simmer for about 2 minutes, or until the sauce is thick and reduced. Taste for seasoning and add more soy sauce or chilli sauce if liked.

4 Add the bean sprouts and toss vigorously to mix all the ingredients together, sprinkle with the pomegranate seeds and serve immediately.

stir-fried pork with tofu and mangetout

Serves 3 – Preparation time: 15–20 minutes – Cooking time: about 15 minutes

Per serving – Energy 416 kcals/1734 kJ · Protein 39 g · Carbohydrate 11 g · Fat 25 g · Saturated fat 6 g · Fibre 2 g

3	**tablespoons groundnut oil**
375 g	**(12 oz) pork fillet (tenderloin), cut into thin strips against the grain**
250–300 g	**(8–10 oz) firm tofu, drained, dried and cut into cubes**
125 g	**(4 oz) mangetout, trimmed**
2	**garlic cloves, crushed**
250 g	**(8 oz) Chinese cabbage, shredded pepper**
1	**teaspoon sesame oil, to finish**

Sauce:

2	**teaspoons cornflour**
6	**tablespoons chicken stock or water**
3	**tablespoons soy sauce**
2	**tablespoons Chinese rice wine or dry sherry**
½	**teaspoon Chinese five-spice powder**
¼	**teaspoon chilli powder, or to taste**

alcohol free	
citrus free	✔
dairy free	✔
gluten free	
wheat free	

1 First prepare the sauce. Blend the cornflour to a paste with 2 tablespoons of the stock or water, then stir in the remaining stock or water and the rest of the sauce ingredients.

2 Heat an empty wok until hot. Add 2 tablespoons of the groundnut oil and heat until hot. Add the pork strips and stir-fry over a high heat for 3–4 minutes or until lightly coloured on all sides. Remove the wok from the heat and tip the pork and its juices into a bowl.

3 Return the wok to a moderate heat. Add the remaining groundnut oil and heat until hot. Add the tofu and stir-fry for 1–2 minutes or until lightly coloured on all sides. Remove the wok from the heat and transfer the tofu to kitchen paper with a slotted spoon. Keep hot.

4 Return the wok to the heat and add the mangetout and garlic. Stir-fry for 2 minutes. Return the pork and its juices to the wok, add the Chinese cabbage and stir-fry for 30 seconds, just until mixed with the pork and mangetout.

5 Stir the sauce to mix, then pour it into the wok. Increase the heat to high and stir for 1–2 minutes or until the sauce thickens. Gently fold in the tofu. Add pepper to taste and sprinkle with the sesame oil. Serve immediately.

sweet and sour pork

Serves 3 – Preparation time: 15 minutes – Cooking time: 15 minutes

Per serving – Energy 519 kcals/2178 kJ · Protein 22 g · Carbohydrate 54 g · Fat 24 g · Saturated fat 4 g · Fibre 2 g

alcohol free	
citrus free	✔
dairy free	✔
gluten free	
wheat free	

250 g (8 oz) pork, cut into cubes
1 teaspoon salt
1½ tablespoons brandy
1 egg, beaten
1 tablespoon cornflour
vegetable oil for deep-frying
125 g (4 oz) bamboo shoots, cut into chunks
1 green pepper, cored, deseeded and
cut into chunks
2 spring onions, cut into 2.5 cm
(1 inch) lengths
425 g (14 oz) can pineapple chunks in juice,
drained and juice reserved

Sauce:
3 tablespoons vinegar
3 tablespoons sugar
½ teaspoon salt
1 tablespoon tomato purée
1 tablespoon soy sauce
1 tablespoon cornflour
1 teaspoon sesame oil

1 Place the pork in a bowl and sprinkle with the salt and brandy. Marinate in the refrigerator for 15 minutes. Add the beaten egg and cornflour and blend well.

2 Heat the oil in a wok to 180–190°C (350–375°F). Remove the wok from the heat but leave the pork in the oil for a further 2 minutes, then remove with a slotted spoon and drain on kitchen paper. Return the wok to the heat and reheat the pork with the bamboo shoots for 2 minutes. Remove and drain on kitchen paper.

3 Pour off the excess oil, leaving 1 tablespoonful in the wok. Add the green pepper and spring onions. Mix all the sauce ingredients with a little canned pineapple juice and add to the wok, stirring until thickened. Add the pork, bamboo shoots and pineapple chunks and serve hot.

pork and vegetables

Serves 3 – Preparation time: 15 minutes – Cooking time: 8–10 minutes

Per serving – Energy 397 kcals/1653 kJ · Protein 22 g · Carbohydrate 20 g · Fat 25 g · Saturated fat 4 g · Fibre 6

alcohol free	
citrus free	✔
dairy free	✔
gluten free	
wheat free	

2 tablespoons soy sauce
1 tablespoon dry sherry
2 teaspoons cornflour
250 g (8 oz) pork fillet, thinly sliced
5 tablespoons vegetable oil
2 spring onions, cut into 2.5 cm
(1 inch) lengths
1 slice root ginger, finely chopped
125 g (4 oz) fresh bean sprouts
1 small green pepper, cored,
deseeded and sliced
a few cauliflower or broccoli florets
2–3 tomatoes, cut into pieces
2 carrots, cut into pieces
50 g (2 oz) green beans, trimmed
2 teaspoons salt
1 tablespoon sugar
3 tablespoons chicken stock or water
rice, to serve

1 Mix together the soy sauce, sherry and cornflour in a bowl, and add the pork. Stir well until each slice is coated with the mixture.

2 Heat half of the oil in a wok. Add the sliced pork and stir-fry for 1 minute, then remove with a slotted spoon and set aside.

3 Heat the remaining oil and add the spring onions and ginger, followed by the bean sprouts, green pepper, cauliflower or broccoli, tomatoes, carrots, green beans, salt and sugar. Stir-fry for 1–2 minutes and then add the sliced pork. Moisten with a little stock or water if prefered and stir-fry quickly until the vegetables are tender but still crisp. Serve immediately with rice.

beef with broccoli and oyster sauce

Serves 2 – Preparation time: about 15 minutes (plus freezing and marinating) **– Cooking time: 15–20 minutes**

Per serving – Energy 486 kcals/2040 kJ · Protein 52 g · Carbohydrate 26 g · Fat 20 g · Saturated fat 6 g · Fibre 3 g

1	piece of rump steak, weighing about 375 g (12 oz), trimmed of all fat
1	egg white
2	tablespoons soy sauce
2	garlic cloves, crushed
2.5 cm	(1 inch) piece of root ginger, grated
1	tablespoon cornflour
1	teaspoon sugar
	about 50 ml (2 fl oz) groundnut oil, for frying
250 g	(8 oz) broccoli, divided into small florets
125 ml	(4 fl oz) Chinese rice wine or dry sherry
3	tablespoons oyster sauce
2	tablespoons soy sauce, or more to taste
	salt and pepper

To Garnish.
	sesame oil
2	tablespoons toasted sesame seeds small bunch of chives, snipped (optional)

1 Wrap the beef in clingfilm and put it in the freezer for 1–2 hours until it is just hard.

2 Remove the beef from the freezer and unwrap it, then slice it into rectangles about the size of a large postage stamp, working against the grain. Whisk the egg white in a non-metallic dish, add the soy sauce, garlic, ginger, cornflour and sugar and whisk to mix. Add the beef, stir to coat, then leave to marinate at room temperature for about 30 minutes or until the beef is completely thawed out.

3 Heat the oil in a wok until very hot, but not smoking. Add about one-third of the beef rectangles and stir them around so they separate. Fry for 30–60 seconds until the beef changes colour all over, lift out with a slotted spoon and drain on kitchen paper. Repeat with the remaining beef. Very carefully pour off all but about 2 tablespoons of the hot oil from the wok.

4 Add the broccoli florets to the wok, sprinkle with the rice wine or sherry and toss over a moderate heat for 3 minutes. Return the beef to the wok and add the oyster sauce and soy sauce. Increase the heat to high and stir-fry vigorously for 3–4 minutes or until the beef and broccoli are tender. Taste for seasoning, and add more soy sauce if liked. Serve hot, drizzled with a little sesame oil and sprinkled with toasted sesame seeds. Garnish with snipped chives, if liked.

alcohol free	
citrus free	✔
dairy free	✔
gluten free	
wheat free	

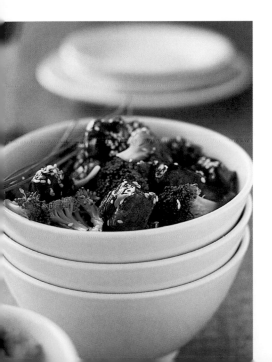

chinese minced beef with tofu

Serves 2 – Preparation time: 10 minutes – Cooking time: about 10 minutes

Per serving – Energy 404 kcals/1685 kJ · Protein 28 g · Carbohydrate 16 g · Fat 26 g · Saturated fat 5 g · Fibre 1 g

✔ alcohol free
✔ citrus free
✔ dairy free
✔ gluten free
✔ wheat free

2   **teaspoons cornflour**
150 ml   **(¼ pint) cold water**
2   **tablespoons soy sauce**
2   **tablespoons hoisin sauce**
2   **teaspoons chilli sauce**
1   **teaspoon dark soft brown sugar**
2   **tablespoons groundnut oil**
125 g   **(4 oz) minced beef**
2   **teaspoons black bean sauce**
6   **button mushrooms,**
     quartered lengthways
4   **spring onions, thinly sliced into rings**
3   **garlic cloves, crushed**
300 g   **(10 oz) tofu, drained, dried and diced**
1   **tablespoon sesame oil**

To Serve:
½–1   **teaspoon chilli oil, to taste**
     rice noodles (optional)

1   Blend the cornflour in a jug with 50 ml (2 fl oz) of the cold water, then add the remaining cold water, the soy, hoisin and chilli sauces and the sugar. Stir well to combine.

2   Heat an empty wok until hot. Add the oil and heat. Add the meat and black bean sauce, the mushrooms and half of the spring onions. Stir-fry over a high heat for 3–4 minutes. Add the garlic, the cornflour mixture and tofu and bring to the boil, stirring until thickened and glossy. Stir-fry for a further 2 minutes, then sprinkle with the remaining spring onions and the sesame oil. Serve drizzled with chilli oil to taste, accompanied by rice noodles if liked.

paper-thin lamb with garlic and spring onions

Serves 3 – Preparation time: 10 minutes, plus freezing – Cooking time: about 6 minutes

Per serving – Energy 364 kcals/1519 kJ · Protein 35 g · Carbohydrate 3 g · Fat 24 g · Saturated fat 8 g · Fibre 1 g

alcohol free
✔ citrus free
✔ dairy free
gluten free
wheat free

500 g   **(1 lb) lamb neck fillet, trimmed of fat**
     and sinew
2   **tablespoons groundnut oil**
3   **large garlic cloves, thinly sliced**
½   **teaspoon chilli powder, or to taste**
½   **teaspoon dark soft brown sugar**
     pinch of salt
1   **large bunch of spring onions,**
     cut into 7 cm (3 inch) lengths
     and shredded lengthways
2   **tablespoons soy sauce**
2   **tablespoons Chinese rice wine**
     or dry sherry
2   **teaspoons sesame oil**

1   Wrap the lamb in clingfilm and put it in the freezer for 1–2 hours until just hard. Cut it into paper-thin slices against the grain. Leave at room temperature for about 30 minutes or until completely thawed out.

2   Add the groundnut oil to a hot wok and heat. Add the garlic and stir-fry over a low heat for a few seconds to flavour the oil, then add the lamb and sprinkle with the chilli powder, sugar and salt. Increase the heat to high and stir-fry for 3–4 minutes until the lamb is browned.

3   Add the spring onions, soy sauce and rice wine or sherry and stir-fry for 30–60 seconds or until all the ingredients are quite dry. Serve immediately, sprinkled with the sesame oil.

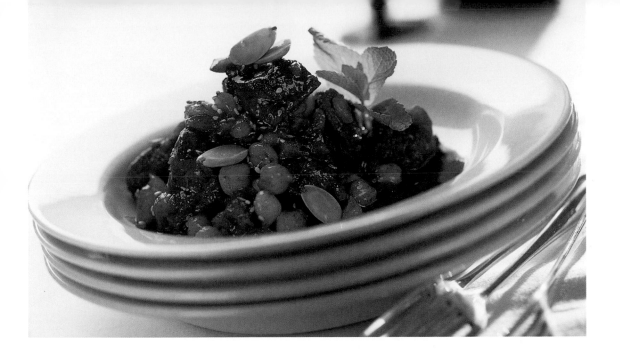

moroccan lamb

Serves 4 – Preparation time: 15 minutes, plus soaking – Cooking time: about 2½ hours

Per serving – Energy 622 kcals/2615 kJ · Protein 45 g · Carbohydrate 52 g · Fat 28 g · Saturated fat 7 g · Fibre 12 g

250 g	(8 oz) chickpeas, soaked overnight
75 g	(3 oz) dried apricots, soaked overnight
2	tablespoons vegetable oil
500 g	(1 lb) lean, boneless lamb, cut into 1 cm (½ inch) cubes
1	large onion, chopped
1	garlic clove, crushed
300 ml	(½ pint) chicken stock
2	tablespoons clear honey
1	teaspoon ground cinnamon
½	teaspoon ground allspice
½	teaspoon cumin seeds
	very finely pared rind of ½ orange
	salt and pepper

To Garnish:

50 g	(2 oz) halved almonds, fried or toasted
1	tablespoon sesame seeds, toasted
	mint sprigs

1 Drain the chickpeas. Drain the soaked apricots and cut them into small pieces. Heat 1 tablespoon of the oil in a flameproof casserole and fry the lamb until lightly browned and sealed all over. Remove from the casserole with a slotted spoon and set aside.

2 Add the remaining oil, the onion and garlic to the casserole and fry very gently for about 5 minutes until soft. Add the stock and stir well.

3 Return the meat to the casserole and stir in the drained chickpeas. Cover closely with a lid or foil and cook on the centre shelf of a preheated oven, 160°C (325°F), Gas Mark 3, for 1 hour.

4 Add the honey, cinnamon, allspice, cumin seeds, orange rind and apricots and stir well together. Cover the casserole and return it to the oven for a further 1–1½ hours, or until the lamb is tender. Discard the orange rind.

5 Transfer the lamb to warm plates. Scatter over the almonds over the top, sprinkle with sesame seeds and top with mint sprigs.

alcohol free	✔
citrus free	
dairy free	✔
gluten free	✔
wheat free	✔

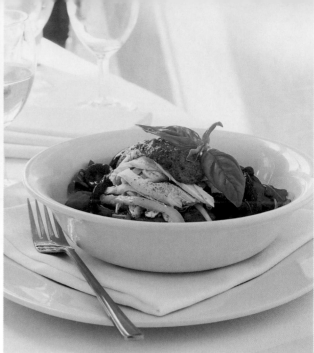
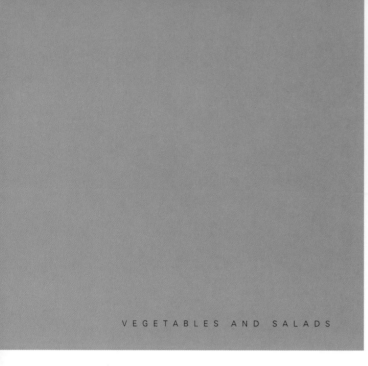

VEGETABLES AND SALADS

pesto chicken and pepper salad

Serves 4 – Preparation time: 20 minutes – Cooking time: 20 minutes

Per serving – Energy 329 kcals/1372 kJ · Protein 33 g · Carbohydrate 3 g · Fat 21 g · Saturated fat 5 g · Fibre 2 g

✔	alcohol free
✔	citrus free
	dairy free
✔	gluten free
✔	wheat free

1 **small cooked chicken**
1 **red pepper**
1 **yellow pepper**
75 g **(3 oz) mixed salad leaves (such as rocket, frisée, young spinach)**
50 g **(2 oz) black olives, pitted**
olive oil, to drizzle
salt and pepper
basil sprigs, to garnish

Pesto Dressing:
15 g **(½ oz) basil leaves**
15 g **(½ oz) Parmesan cheese, grated**
2 **tablespoons white wine vinegar**
½ **tablespoon pine nuts**
1 **small garlic clove, crushed**
50 ml **(2 fl oz) extra virgin olive oil**

1 Skin the chicken and remove all the meat from the carcass. Shred the meat and set aside.

2 Cook the peppers under a preheated hot grill for 15–20 minutes, turning occasionally, until the skin is blistered and blackened all over. Transfer the peppers to a plastic bag and set aside to cool.

3 To make the pesto dressing, put the basil, Parmesan, vinegar, pine nuts and garlic into a food processor or blender, add pepper to taste and purée for a few seconds. With the motor running, drizzle the olive oil through the feeder tube until the mixture becomes thick and smooth.

4 When the peppers are cool enough to handle, rub off and discard the charred skin. Slice the flesh into thin strips, and discard the seeds and core. Season with salt and pepper.

5 Arrange the salad leaves in bowls. Pile the peppers on to the salad leaves, with the olives and chicken. Spoon the pesto over the chicken mixture. Serve immediately, drizzled with olive oil and garnished with basil sprigs.

japanese seaweed salad

Serves 4 – Preparation time: 5–10 minutes, plus softening – Cooking time: 5 minutes

Per serving – Energy 50 kcals/215 kJ · Protein 4 g · Carbohydrate 10 g · Fat 0 g · Saturated fat 0 g · Fibre 3 g

25 g	(1 oz) mixed dried seaweed,
	such as dulse or sea lettuce
	wedges of lime or lemon, to serve

Mirin Dressing:

75 ml	(3 fl oz) mirin
	(sweet Japanese rice wine)
75 ml	(3 fl oz) rice wine vinegar
75 ml	(3 fl oz) dashi (see page 75)
2	tablespoons caster sugar

1 Place the seaweed in a bowl, cover with cold water and leave for 15 minutes to soften.

2 To make the dressing, mix the mirin, vinegar and dashi in a small saucepan with the sugar and heat gently until the sugar has dissolved. Remove from the heat and leave to cool.

3 When the seaweed is soft, drain it well and arrange it on individual plates. Dress with the mirin dresing. Serve with wedges of lime or lemon to squeeze over the seaweed.

alcohol free	
citrus free	
dairy free	✔
gluten free	✔
wheat free	✔

roasted beetroot citrus salad

Serves 6 – Preparation time: 20 minutes – Cooking time: 35 minutes

Per serving – Energy 117 kcals/484 kJ · Protein 2 g · Carbohydrate 12 g · Fat: 7 g · Saturated fat 1 g · Fibre 2 g

6	beetroots, peeled and halved
4	Spanish onions, halved
50 ml	(2 fl oz) olive oil
75 ml	(3 fl oz) balsamic vinegar

Dressing:

1	tablespoon finely grated orange rind
50 ml	(2 fl oz) fresh orange juice
50 ml	(2 fl oz) olive oil
50 ml	(2 fl oz) balsamic vinegar

1 Arrange the halved beetroots and onions in a single layer in an ovenproof dish. Mix together the oil and vinegar and pour it over the beetroots and onions. Bake in a preheated oven, 200°C (400°F), Gas Mark 6, for 35 minutes or until the beetroots are just tender. Transfer the beetroots and onions to a serving dish.

2 To make the dressing, place the orange rind in a bowl with the orange juice, oil and vinegar, and whisk to combine.

3 Pour the dressing over the beetroots and onions and serve immediately.

alcohol free	✔
citrus free	
dairy free	✔
gluten free	✔
wheat free	✔

three-bean fusilli salad

Serves 4 – Preparation time: 20 minutes – Cooking time: about 12 minutes

Per serving – Energy 420 kcals/1780 kJ · Protein 16 g · Carbohydrate 71 g · Fat 10 g · Saturated fat 6 g · Fibre 8 g

✔ alcohol free
✔ citrus free
dairy free
gluten free
wheat free

oil, see method
300 g (10 oz) dried tricolore fusilli
2 spring onions, chopped diagonally
**1 red pepper, cored, deseeded
    and chopped**
125 g (4 oz) drained canned red kidney beans
125 g (4 oz) drained canned pinto beans
125 g (4 oz) drained canned borlotti beans
200 ml (7 fl oz) half-fat crème fraîche
4 tablespoons milk
3 tablespoons chopped dill
salt and pepper
dill sprigs, to garnish

1 Bring at least 1.8 litres (3 pints) water to the boil in a large saucepan. Add a dash of oil and a generous pinch of salt. Cook the pasta for 8–12 minutes, until just tender. Drain then rinse under cold water in a colander, drain again and transfer to a large salad bowl.

2 Add the spring onions, red pepper and beans. Mix well. Beat together the crème fraîche and milk in a bowl; fold into the salad and add salt and pepper to taste. Fold in the chopped dill, garnish with dill sprigs and serve.

sichuan tofu

Serves 4 – Preparation time: 15 minutes, plus soaking – Cooking time: about 15 minutes

Per serving – Energy 147 kcals/613 kJ · Protein 8 g · Carbohydrate 8 g · Fat 9 g · Saturated fat 2 g · Fibre 1 g

alcohol free
✔ citrus free
✔ dairy free
✔ gluten free
✔ wheat free

6 dried shiitake mushrooms
125 ml (4 fl oz) hot water
2 tablespoons groundnut oil
**4 spring onions, cut crossways
    into quarters**
**1 small red pepper, cored,
    deseeded and finely diced**
**1 small green pepper, cored,
    deseeded and finely diced**
2 garlic cloves, finely chopped
**1 bird's eye chilli, deseeded and
    very finely chopped**
**2 heaped tablespoons canned salted black
    beans, rinsed and coarsely mashed**
2 tablespoons black bean sauce
**2 tablespoons Chinese rice wine
    or dry sherry**
4 tablespoons cold water
**300 g (10 oz) firm tofu, drained, dried and cut
    into 2.5–4 cm (1–1½ inch) squares**
salt and pepper
chilli oil, to finish

1 Soak the dried mushrooms in the hot water for 35–40 minutes. Drain the mushrooms in a sieve over a bowl and reserve the soaking water. Cut the mushroom caps into small squares, discarding any hard stalks.

2 Heat an empty wok until hot. Add the oil and heat until hot. Add the spring onions, red and green peppers, garlic, chilli and mushrooms, stir-fry for 1–2 minutes, then add the black beans and black bean sauce, the rice wine or sherry, the mushroom soaking liquid and the cold water. Bring to the boil and simmer for 5 minutes, then add the tofu and stir gently to mix. Simmer for another 5 minutes, stirring occasionally. Taste for seasoning and serve hot, drizzled with chilli oil.

crispy seaweed

Serves 8 – Preparation time: 10 minutes, plus drying – Cooking time: 10 minutes

Per serving – Energy 70 kcals/293 kJ · Protein 3 g · Carbohydrate 4 g · Fat 5 g · Saturated fat 1 g · Fibre 6 g

750 g	(1½ lb) spring greens, finely shredded
	vegetable oil, for deep-frying
1½	teaspoons caster sugar
1	teaspoon salt

1 Spread out the shredded spring greens on kitchen paper for about 30 minutes until thoroughly dry.

2 Heat the oil in a wok to 180–190°C (350–375°F). Turn off the heat for 30 seconds and then add a small batch of shredded spring greens. Turn up the heat to moderate and deep-fry the greens until they begin to float on the surface of the oil. Take care, as they tend to spit while they are cooking.

3 Remove the greens with a slotted spoon and drain on kitchen paper. Cook the remaining greens in batches in the same way. When they are all cooked, transfer to a bowl and sprinkle over the sugar and salt. Toss gently to mix and serve warm or cold with Chinese dishes.

alcohol free	✔
citrus free	✔
dairy free	✔
gluten free	✔
wheat free	✔

green beans with broccoli and almonds

Serves 4 – Preparation time: 10–15 minutes – Cooking time: about 12 minutes

Per serving – Energy 170 kcals/707 kJ · Protein 6 g · Carbohydrate 7 g · Fat 13 g · Saturated fat 2 g · Fibre 3 g

2	teaspoons cornflour
6	tablespoons vegetable stock or water
2	tablespoons soy sauce
1	tablespoon lemon juice
4	tablespoons flaked almonds
2	tablespoons groundnut oil
175 g	(6 oz) broccoli, separated into
	small florets
175 g	(6 oz) green beans, cut diagonally
	into 4–5 cm (1½–2 inch lengths)
3	garlic cloves, crushed
	pepper

1 Blend the cornflour in a jug with 2 tablespoons of the stock or water, then add the remaining stock or water and the soy sauce and lemon juice. Stir well to combine.

2 Dry-fry the flaked almonds in a wok over a moderate heat for 1–2 minutes until lightly toasted, then remove them and set aside.

3 Heat the oil in the wok until hot, add the broccoli and stir-fry for 3 minutes. Add the beans and garlic and stir-fry for 3–4 minutes.

4 Pour in the cornflour mixture and bring to the boil over a high heat, stirring constantly until thickened. Add pepper to taste and serve sprinkled with the almonds.

alcohol free	✔
citrus free	
dairy free	✔
gluten free	
wheat free	

steamed vegetables with ginger

Serves 4 – Preparation time: 10 minutes – Cooking time: 7 minutes

Per serving – Energy 54 kcals/226 kJ · Protein 3 g · Carbohydrate 9 g · Fat 1 g · Saturated fat 0 g · Fibre 2 g

✔ alcohol free
✔ citrus free
✔ dairy free
✔ gluten free
✔ wheat free

3   carrots, cut into 5 mm (¼ inch) rounds
75 g   (3 oz) cauliflower florets
75 g   (3 oz) broccoli florets
2   small courgettes, cut into
1 cm (½ inch) rounds
3.5 cm   (1½ inch) piece root ginger,
cut into thin strips

1 Place all the vegetables in a steamer with the ginger and steam over boiling water for 7 minutes until tender.

caponata

Serves 6 – Preparation time: 20 minutes, plus standing – Cooking time: about 1¼ hours

Per serving – Energy 83 kcals/347 kJ · Protein 3 g · Carbohydrate 5 g · Fat 6 g · Saturated fat 1 g · Fibre 3 g

✔ alcohol free
✔ citrus free
✔ dairy free
✔ gluten free
✔ wheat free

3   aubergines, cut into 1 cm (½ inch) dice
2   tablespoons olive oil
1   onion, thinly sliced
2   celery sticks, diced
150 ml   (¼ pint) passata
(Italian chopped tomatoes)
3   tablespoons wine vinegar
1   yellow pepper, cored, deseeded
and thinly sliced
1   red pepper, cored, deseeded
and thinly sliced
25 g   (1 oz) anchovy fillets, soaked
in warm water, drained and dried
50 g   (2 oz) capers, roughly chopped
25 g   (1 oz) black olives, pitted and sliced
25 g   (1 oz) green olives, pitted and sliced
salt
2   tablespoons chopped parsley, to serve

1 Put the diced aubergines into a colander, sprinkle with salt and leave to drain for 15–20 minutes to exude their bitter juices. Rinse under cold running water to remove any salt and pat dry with kitchen paper.

2 Heat the oil in a saucepan, add the onion and sauté until soft and golden. Add the celery and cook for 2–3 minutes. Add the aubergine and cook gently for 3 minutes, stirring occasionally. Add the passata and cook gently until it has been absorbed. Add the wine vinegar and cook for 1 minute. Add the peppers, anchovies, capers and olives and cook for 3 minutes.

3 Transfer the mixture to an ovenproof dish and bake, covered, in a preheated oven, 180°C (350°F), Gas Mark 4, for about 1 hour. Serve lukewarm or cold, sprinkled with chopped parsley.

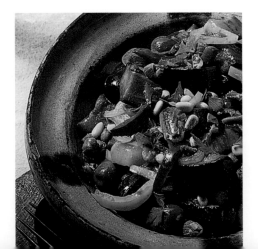

stir-fried mixed vegetables

Serves 4 – Preparation time: 15 minutes – Cooking time: 6–7 minutes

Per serving – Energy 137 kcals/569 kJ · Protein 5 g · Carbohydrate 9 g · Fat 10 g · Saturated fat 1 g · Fibre 4 g

3	tablespoons vegetable oil
1	garlic clove, crushed
125 g	(4 oz) cabbage, shredded
125 g	(4 oz) cauliflower, divided into florets
125 g	(4 oz) broccoli, divided into florets
½	teaspoon pepper
2	tablespoons oyster sauce
150 ml	(¼ pint) chicken or vegetable stock
2	carrots, cut into matchstick strips
125 g	(4 oz) mushrooms, thinly sliced
1	onion, sliced
50 g	(2 oz) bean sprouts

1 Heat the oil in a wok. Add the crushed garlic and stir-fry quickly over moderate heat until golden. Do not let it get too brown.

2 Add the shredded cabbage, cauliflower, broccoli, and the black pepper. Stir in the oyster sauce and the chicken or vegetable stock and then cook, stirring constantly, for 3 minutes.

3 Add the carrots, mushrooms and onion to the wok together with the bean sprouts. Stir-fry for 2 minutes. Transfer the fried vegetables to a large dish or platter and serve immediately.

alcohol free	✔
citrus free	✔
dairy free	✔
gluten free	✔
wheat free	✔

chinese braised vegetables

Serves 4 – Preparation time: 20 minutes – Cooking time: 15 minutes

Per serving – Energy 223 kcals/929 kJ · Protein 9 g · Carbohydrate 14 g · Fat 15 g · Saturated fat 2 g · Fibre 2 g

5–6	Chinese dried mushrooms, soaked in warm water for 20 minutes
250 g	(8 oz) firm tofu, cut into cubes
4	tablespoons vegetable oil
125 g	(4 oz) carrots, sliced
125 g	(4 oz) mangetout, trimmed
125 g	(4 oz) Chinese leaves, shredded
2	spring onions, cut into 1 cm (½ inch) lengths
125 g	(4 oz) bamboo shoots, sliced
1	teaspoon sugar
1	tablespoon light soy sauce
1	teaspoon cornflour
1	tablespoon cold water
1	teaspoon sesame oil
	salt

1 Drain the dried mushrooms and squeeze them dry. Discard the hard stalks and cut the caps into thin slices.

2 Bring a saucepan of lightly salted water to the boil and add the tofu. Boil for 2–3 minutes until firm. Remove the tofu pieces with a slotted spoon and drain well on kitchen paper.

3 Heat about half of the oil in a wok. Add the tofu and fry until lightly browned. Remove with a slotted spoon and set aside. Heat the remaining oil in the wok. Add the vegetables and stir-fry for 2 minutes. Stir in the tofu with 1 teaspoon salt, the sugar and soy sauce. Cover, reduce the heat and braise for 3 minutes.

4 Meanwhile, mix the cornflour to a smooth paste with the water. Stir into the braised vegetables in the wok. Increase the heat and continue stirring until the sauce thickens. Sprinkle in the sesame oil and serve immediately.

alcohol free	✔
citrus free	✔
dairy free	✔
gluten free	
wheat free	

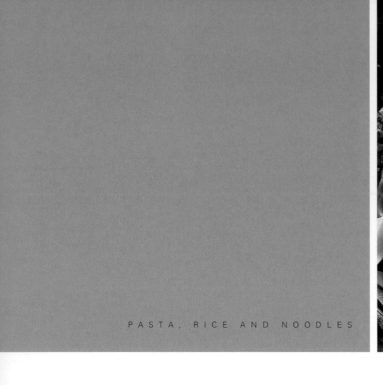
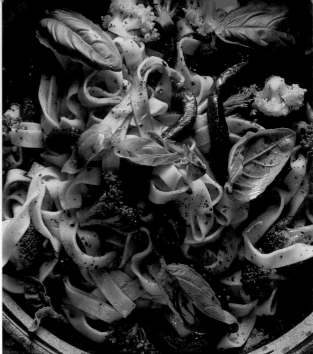

broccoli and red pepper fettuccine salad

Serves 4 – Preparation time: 10 minutes – Cooking time: about 15 minutes

Per serving – Energy 375 kcals/1510 kJ · Protein 13 g · Carbohydrate 51 g · Fat 14 g · Saturated fat 2 g · Fibre 1 g

✔	alcohol free
✔	citrus free
✔	dairy free
	gluten free
	wheat free

4	**tablespoons olive oil**
300 g	**(10 oz) fresh fettuccine**
3	**red peppers, cored,**
	deseeded and halved
250 g	**(8 oz) small broccoli florets**
2	**tablespoons balsamic vinegar**
	salt and pepper
	basil leaves, to garnish

1 Bring at least 1.8 litres (3 pints) water to the boil in a large saucepan. Add a dash of oil and a pinch of salt. Cook the pasta for 4–6 minutes, until just tender. Drain, rinse under cold running water in a colander and drain again. Set aside in a large salad bowl.

2 Grill the peppers, skin side up, until the skins have blackened and blistered. Remove from the heat and leave to cool for 5 minutes.

3 Meanwhile, bring a large saucepan of lightly salted water to the boil and blanch the broccoli florets for 3 minutes. Drain, rinse under cold running water and drain again.

4 Peel the peppers and slice the flesh into strips. Add to the pasta with the drained broccoli florets, the remaining olive oil and the balsamic vinegar. Add salt and pepper to taste and toss well. Serve immediately, garnished with basil leaves.

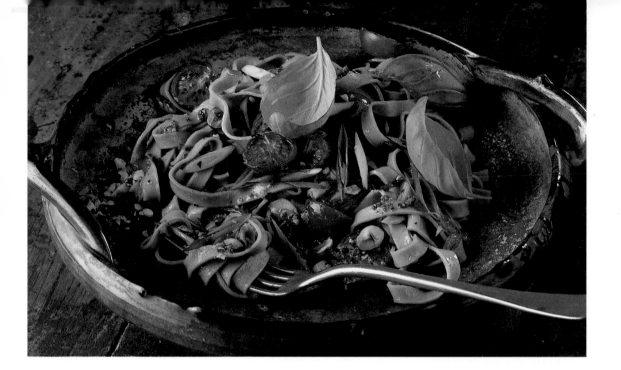

tagliatelle with chilli and roast cherry tomato dressing

Serves 4 – Preparation time: 10 minutes – Cooking time: 15 minutes

Per serving – Energy 574 kcals/2305 kJ · Protein 18 g · Carbohydrate 79 g · Fat 21 g · Saturated fat 3 g · Fibre 2 g

250 g	(8 oz) cherry tomatoes
2	teaspoons ready-made pesto
4	tablespoons olive oil, plus a dash
2	spring onions, thinly sliced
1	red or green chilli, deseeded and finely chopped
2	garlic cloves, chopped
1	tablespoon raspberry vinegar
1	tablespoon orange juice
2	tablespoons toasted hazelnuts, chopped
2	tablespoons chopped basil
500 g	(1 lb) fresh tagliatelle verde
	salt and pepper
	a few basil leaves, to garnish

1 Halve the tomatoes and arrange them on a baking sheet. Sprinkle with a little salt and top with pesto. Toss carefully, making sure you coat the tomatoes well. Cook in a pre-heated oven, 200°C (400°F), Gas Mark 6, for 15 minutes.

2 Meanwhile, heat the olive oil in a small saucepan. Add the spring onions, chilli and garlic and fry for 1 minute, stirring continuously. Remove from the heat, add the vinegar, orange juice, hazelnuts and basil. Stir well, season with salt and pepper and keep warm.

3 Meanwhile, bring at least 1.8 litres (3 pints) water to the boil in a large saucepan. Add a dash of oil and a generous pinch of salt. Just before the tomatoes are ready, cook the pasta for 4 minutes or according to the packet instructions. Drain the pasta and return it to the pan. Add the spring onion mixture and toss well. Add the tomatoes and all the cooking juices. Serve garnished with basil.

alcohol free	✔
citrus free	
dairy free	✔
gluten free	
wheat free	

spaghetti with marinated vegetables

Serves 4 – Preparation time: 20 minutes, plus chilling – Cooking time: 25 minutes

Per serving – Energy 480 kcals/2015 kJ · Protein 11 g · Carbohydrate 59 g · Fat 24 g · Saturated fat 3 g · Fibre 7 g

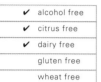

✔	alcohol free
✔	citrus free
✔	dairy free
	gluten free
	wheat free

1	**red pepper, halved, cored and deseeded**
1	**tablespoon salt**
1	**small aubergine, sliced**
125 g	**(4 oz) flat field mushrooms**
1	**leek, trimmed, cleaned and thinly sliced**
1	**teaspoon cumin seeds**
½	**teaspoon coriander seeds**
150 ml	**(¼ pint) raspberry vinegar**
8	**tablespoons olive oil**
1	**tablespoon garlic purée**
300 g	**(10 oz) dried spaghetti**
	salt and pepper

To Garnish:
mixed salad leaves
flat leaf parsley

1 Place the red pepper halves on a grill pan, skin side up, and grill under a high heat for about 10 minutes until the skin is blackened and blistered. Remove from the heat and leave to cool.

2 Meanwhile, sprinkle the salt over the aubergine slices and set aside for 15 minutes. Drain the aubergine slices, rinse them well and pat dry with kitchen paper. Place on a grill pan, and grill under a high heat for 10 minutes, turning the slices once, until browned. Remove from the grill pan and set aside. Add the mushrooms to the grill pan and grill for 2 minutes.

3 Peel the pepper and finely slice the flesh. Slice the mushrooms. Combine all the grilled vegetables in a large bowl and add the leek. Stir in the spices, vinegar, oil and garlic purée with salt and pepper to taste. Toss the mixture until combined, and set aside.

4 Bring at least 1.8 litres (3 pints) water to the boil in a large saucepan. Add a dash of oil and a generous pinch of salt. Cook the pasta for 8–12 minutes, until just tender. Drain thoroughly and add to the vegetable mixture. Toss again and chill for 3 hours before serving.

5 Serve garnished with salad leaves and flat leaf parsley.